46 DAYS

To Sandka —

46 DAYS

Keeping Up with Jennifer Pharr Davis
on the Appalachian Trail

BREW DAVIS

Foreword by
Jennifer Pharr Davis

Jennifer Pharr Davis

BEAUFORT BOOKS • NEW YORK

Library of Congress Cataloging-in-Publication Data

Davis, Brew.

46 days : keeping up with Jennifer Pharr Davis on the Appalachian Trail / Brew Davis
with Jennifer Pharr Davis.

p. cm.

ISBN 978-0-8253-0678-5 (alk. paper)

1. Hiking—Appalachian Trail. 2. Backpacking—Appalachian Trail. I. Pharr Davis,
Jennifer II. Title.

GV199.42.A68D37 2011

796.510974—dc23

2011043243

For inquiries about volume orders, please contact:
Beaufort Books
27 West 20th Street, Suite 1102
New York, NY 10011
sales@beaufortbooks.com

Published in the United States by Beaufort Books
www.beaufortbooks.com

Distributed by Midpoint Trade Books
www.midpointtrade.com

Interior design by Neuwirth & Associates, Inc.

10 9 8 7 6 5 4 3 2 1

Printed in the United States of America

May your trails be crooked, winding, lonesome, dangerous, leading to the most amazing view. May your mountains rise into and above the clouds.

Earth Apples: The Poetry of Edward Abbey (1994)

First to my wonderful wife.
Then to the Pit Crew, who helped her to do something amazing.

CONTENTS

Listening and Following, by Jennifer Pharr Davis   xiii

Introduction   xvii

Frequently Asked Questions about the 2011 Record   xxiii

DAY 1: *56 miles*   1

DAY 2: *44 miles*   3

DAY 3: *46 miles*   5

DAY 4: *42 miles*   7

DAY 5: *41 miles*   11

DAY 6: *38 miles*   13

DAY 7: *31 miles*   15

DAY 8: *34 miles*   19

DAY 9: *30 miles*   21

DAY 10: *38 miles*   23

DAY 11: *43 miles*   27

DAY 12: *36 miles*   31

DAY 13: *42.5 miles*   35

Day 14: *43.5 miles*   39

Day 15: *47.3 miles*   43

Day 16: *48.7 miles*   47

Day 17: *48.3 miles*   51

Day 18: *49 miles*   55

Day 19: *49 miles*   59

Day 20: *45 miles*   63

Day 21: *52.7 miles*   67

Day 22: *48 miles*   71

Day 23: *46.9 miles*   75

Day 24: *53.9 miles*   79

Day 25: *51.9 miles*   81

Day 26: *52.9 miles*   85

Day 27: *50.2 miles*   89

Day 28: *52.1 miles*   93

Day 29: *46.8 miles*   97

Day 30: *52.9 miles*   101

Day 31: *49.7 miles*   105

Day 32: *52.6 miles*   109

Day 33: *46.9 miles*   113

Day 34: *47.3 miles*   117

Day 35: *50.3 miles*   121

Day 36: *49.2 miles*   125

Day 37: *46.9 miles*   129

DAY 38: *49.8 miles*   133

DAY 39: *46.1 miles*   137

DAY 40: *45.5 miles*   141

DAY 41: *47.2 miles*   145

DAY 42: *50.8 miles*   149

DAY 43: *46.3 miles*   153

DAY 44: *48.2 miles*   157

DAY 45: *52.2 miles*   161

DAY 46: *60.2 miles*   165

DAY 47: *36.2 miles*   173

DAY 48: *aka, The 19th Hole*   181

Reflections, by Jennifer Pharr Davis   183

Acknowledgments   187

LISTENING AND FOLLOWING

L ife is filled with voices. On a daily basis we hear the opinions of advertisements, faith groups, politicians, friends,
and family. We constantly process external noise that tells us
what is responsible, what is successful, and what is normal. All
the noise makes it difficult to find silence and the differing
opinions make it difficult to find ourselves.

The most popular question surrounding our 2011 record
attempt on the Appalachian Trail was why? Why would I want
to hike 2,181 miles as fast and efficiently as possible? That, in
itself, is not a difficult question to answer, but it is challenging
to explain.

The simple answer is, that by attempting to set an overall
record on the Appalachian Trail, I was following my heart. I
was listening to the internal voice that screamed in the silence,
filled my head with dreams, and made my stomach feel
uneasy—excited and scared—as if I were on the edge a cliff.
For over two years, my every run, every hike, every lull in the
workday was filled with dreams of the record. I wasn't trying
to think about record, and at some points, I most certainly did
not want to think about record, but its daily presence was
undeniable.

If I had to describe the voice inside that led me back to the
trail, then I would say that it was loud, loud and hopeful. My

reaction to the voice, however, was much different. My response to the swell of possibility within my soul included fear and reason. I was scared I would fail, scared what other people would think, and scared that my husband would resent me for monopolizing another one of "our" summers. I also rationalized that hiking the Appalachian Trail, for the third time, wouldn't prove anything, and it wouldn't put me any closer to the kids and stable income that I wanted to be a part of my future.

But on the trail, I get to leave the noise, erase other people's expectations, and listen to my heart. For me, these silent times of reflection and prayer are found hiking in the woods. I believe that I know who I am standing on top of a mountain, and that I make my best decisions in the heart of the forest. It took ten weeks of backpacking through Europe together before my husband and I made the decision to listen to hope, strip away fear and reason, and try for the overall record on the Appalachian Trail.

The next ten months were filled with training, dreaming, and working on the trail logistics as if they were a Sudoku puzzle. Where could I put in the most miles? Which roads should Brew meet me at? How many calories would I need to consume each day?

It was easy for me to worry that something would go wrong and that we would have to give up the dream before reaching the starting line. I worried that I would get injured or sick. I also worried that something would happen with our jobs or families that would prevent us from hiking. But, most of all, I just tried to enjoy the process. I took my camera on my training excursions and tried to explore trails that I had never been on before. I wondered, after some really hard 30-mile days, how I could average over 45 miles a day for the entire summer. But even when the miles didn't come easily, my training left me feeling reassured in my love for the trail and my desire to try for the overall record.

When my training was finished, and all the details had been addressed, it felt as if, in some way, we had already found success. We believed in ourselves enough to attempt the impossible. Hiking up Katahdin to start the journey, I realized that regardless of what happened on the trail this summer, I would never have to wonder about what could have been.

JENNIFER PHARR DAVIS

INTRODUCTION

———

Jen and I were married on June 8, 2008. Thirteen days later, after honeymooning in Montreal, Montpelier, Vermont, and on the coast of Maine, we camped out at Katahdin Stream Campground and woke up at 3:30 AM to begin hiking up Katahdin.

About a week later, after I'd missed a road crossing near Stratton and the only showers I'd gotten were when our tent leaked during the nightly rain storms, Jen—ever the upbeat thru-hiker—said, "I'm so glad we're out here. This is the perfect way for us to get away from our families and spend time with each other as newlyweds." I sighed loudly and said, "You know, we could have gotten away from our families and spent time together as newlyweds in Fiji instead."

That's kind of been a running joke for us ever since, that and the fact that Jen will owe me for the rest of our lives. After the 2008 hike, she offered to watch 57 Tennessee Titans football games with me—one for every day we spent on the trail—and give me a back massage at every halftime. I, in my wisdom, told her that I didn't want to quantify things, that I'd rather hold it over her for the rest of her life than have it ever come to an end. Now I've supported her on two record attempts so she owes me twice as much. Two life sentences, if you will.

I remember when Jen came up with the idea to return to the trail and go for the overall record. It was spring of 2010. We were walking on the beach near her parents' place at Ocean Isle, North Carolina, when she turned to me nonchalantly and said, "I've been thinking about my AT record . . ." I said, "What have you been thinking?" She said, "Well, I just felt like I had a lot left in the tank when we finished in 2008. Do you think I could have done it faster?" I could already see the wheels turning. I could have squelched her hopes and dreams then and there if I'd just lied to her and told her that I thought she'd maxed out the last time and that she couldn't do it faster. But I remembered how she stopped at 4 PM on Independence Day so we could watch the fireworks and eat funnel cakes in Woodstock, Vermont. How I'd held her up at a road crossing in Pennsylvania because I'd spent too much time at the Yuengling Brewery. Or how Warren and Horton both noted how remarkable she looked toward the end of the hike, how she made 38 miles a day seem almost effortless.

So I had to be honest and tell her, "Yeah, I think you could have done it faster. At least five or six days faster." She replied, "Yeah, that's what I've been thinking, too." She waited for a minute, then said, "So . . . what do you think about us trying to go back and do it again sometime?" And then I knew she had me. She probably knew it, too. Or at least she knew how agreeable I am, that I can't say no to her, that I'm a total pushover. I said, "Honey, if that's what you want to do, then we can talk about it." And just like that, Jen's 2011 Appalachian Trail Record Attempt was on.

Why am I telling you these stories? I'm telling you for two reasons. First, I want to give you some background on Jen's most recent hike. And second, as much as I enjoy living a lie, I want to dispel the myth that I am the perfect husband or some sort of saint.

I'm not. I get cranky a lot. And I got cranky this summer. When Jen wanted to quit near Killington, Vermont, I encouraged her because I genuinely believed she could still break the record. But I also encouraged her because I felt invested. And I guess that's what this summer was really about. Being invested. All in. Together.

For me, being invested meant I didn't allow myself to relax. For almost the entire 46 days, I was a nervous wreck. I knew we had the slimmest of margins and that if I missed Jen at a single road crossing, I could potentially ruin everything. No Yuengling Brewery this time around. Instead, I led this manic existence where I would rush and rush to get to the next road crossing, then, no matter how much I needed to relax or how much free time I really had, I would busy myself with chores—making turkey wraps, organizing the car, or calculating mileage.

I spent hours calculating mileage. How many miles is Jen ahead of Andrew today? How many more miles is she averaging compared to the 2008 hike? How many will she complete if she stops at Bake Oven Road tonight? What was her mile per hour average for the last section? How many miles is she from Delaware Water Gap? How many does she have to Springer?

I told myself that all of the number crunching was to encourage Jen with "positive numbers." And that was true. But it was also because I had a ridiculous amount of nervous energy, and since I had a bum knee, I couldn't get rid of it in a normal, healthy way. So I pored over figures and maps, prepared backpacks, and pretty much did anything to keep myself occupied, including writing blog entries.

I never thought people would enjoy them so much. And I certainly never thought it would turn into a book. I just figured we were doing something cool that our grandkids might want to know about someday, so I decided to keep a somewhat detailed and mildly amusing account.

The other day, I was reading a book by Shane Claiborne called *The Irresistible Revolution*. It's a pretty radical treatise on how Christians have shirked their responsibilities and haven't taken care of the poor. I've read a lot of books about Christianity and I can count on one hand the times that something has struck me to the core. Something Claiborne wrote did that to me the other day. Pretty early in the book, he's talking about miracles, and he writes:

> I started to see that the miracles were an expression not so much of Jesus' mighty power as of his love . . . Jesus raised his friend Lazarus from the dead, and a few years later, Lazarus died again. Jesus healed the sick, but they eventually caught some other disease. He fed the thousands, and the next day they were hungry again. But we remember his love. It wasn't that Jesus healed a leper but that he touched a leper, because no one touched lepers.

Why am I saying that? While Jen and I can be very proud of what we did this summer, it's inevitable that someday, somebody else is going to come along and break Jen's record just like she broke Andrew Thompson's and Andrew Thompson broke Pete Palmer's and Pete Palmer broke David Horton's and so on.

But the deeper miracle or accomplishment or whatever you want to call it is that we went through this ordeal together, that we supported each other wholeheartedly, that we overcame a lot of obstacles, and that through it all, we loved each other really well. I love watching the video clip of us hugging on Springer Mountain because it embodies all of that.

On the surface, that may not be as impressive as setting a record. But in the long run, it's much more significant. I know you may not have chosen to read this book if Jen hadn't broken the record. For that matter, it may not even have been published. But do me a favor and try not to read it just as a journal of a record attempt. Try to read it as a love story. Because that's what it is. And when it's all said and done, love's going to outlast records. Shoot, love's going to outlast everything.

BREW DAVIS

FREQUENTLY ASKED QUESTIONS ABOUT THE 2011 RECORD

———

Why do you want to try for the record?

Because my heart tells me that I should.

When will you start?

Mid June. We will head up to Katahdin and then check out the trail condition and weather before deciding on the exact day.

Why hike Sobo (Southbound)?

It is a great feeling to have Maine and New Hampshire finished at the beginning of the journey. It is also nice to hike home.

Are you posting updates?

Yup. Pics, video, and blogs will periodically appear on Facebook, www.blueridgehikingco.com and Jen's blog.

Are you taking a GPS or Spot or cell phone to track your progress?

No.

Well, how will people know that you are not cheating?

If I wanted to cheat, don't you think I could figure out how to do it with a GPS or Spot? Trail records are based on integrity and a personal honor code. I think that's really cool, and it is one of the reasons I love trail records.

Do the ATC or the NPS recognize trail records?

No, nor should they. I am a member of the Appalachian Trail Conservancy and the last thing I would want my resources spent on is trying to validate trail records. The ATC is doing a great job of protecting, building, and promoting the trail.

How do trail records exist if there isn't an organization that recognizes them?

They don't need to be recognized by an organization; they are acknowledged by the community and held close to the hearts of those who attain them. Setting a trail record is a truly amateur pursuit. There is no reward, t-shirt, or trophy at the end. The people who have set records have sacrificed a great deal personally, financially, relationally. The word amateur comes from the Latin word for love. You HAVE to love the trail to set a trail record.

Okay, but aren't you sponsored?

I have spent my own money to fund over 9,000 miles of hiking on six different continents and volunteered countless hours promoting the trail and long distance hiking. But now that my husband and I are looking toward the future, our yearly hiking fund has become a baby savings account.

I am so thankful that Salomon is supporting me this summer. I used their products before this summer and I truly believe that they are the most performance focused outdoor company. They are providing some amazing shoes and packs, and helping me pay for the endeavor. In fact, because they are helping protect the baby fund, we may consider naming our firstborn son Salomon. Okay, not really, but it is an amazing company and I am "working" for the sponsorship by helping them with a lot of product feedback and development.

Also, I want to give a huge shout-out to my lifelong outfitter in Asheville, Diamond Brand Outdoors. They are providing some yummy Clif Bars, Mountain House, and a lot of love and support! I love you guys!

Do you really think you can break the record?

Yes. I would not have spent the countless hours training and dedicated 7 weeks of my summer to this effort if I didn't believe that I could set the overall record. And I guarantee that my husband would not sacrifice his summer vacation (again) if he didn't believe that I could set the record.

But you're a girl?

Good observation. My previous AT hike in 2008 taught me that setting a record isn't about being fast or strong. It is all about fortitude, intelligence, and perseverance. The fact that women give birth and live longer than guys makes me think that we might even have an evolutionary edge.

Who's helping you on the trail?

Mostly my WONDERFUL husband, Brew. Our good friends Warren Doyle, David Horton, New York Steve, and Melissa will support us through certain sections as well.

Do you feel ready?

Yes. My training went well, and I am just really excited to be on the trail. This doesn't feel out of the ordinary or strange. I have spent the past 8 summers hiking, so my body is screaming at me to get on the trail. I am also VERY ready to stop talking the talk, and just start walking the walk.

So you have an AT book out and a hiking company, is this a well-devised publicity stunt?

There have got to be easier ways to get publicity. This attempt is a calling, passion, and desire. I approached my husband, Warren, and David with this idea well before I had signed a book contract.

Surely you can't enjoy the trail when you are hiking 45 miles a day?

Well, I do. I am not saying that everyone could or would. But I love experiencing the trail in this fashion. There are obviously differences between a record attempt and a thru-hike or section hike. I have said it before, and I will say it again. It is not about how long you are on the trail or how fast you go, it is about what you take from the experience.

So are you running?

Only if I can. It is great when I find a flat stretch or a gentle downhill and my body is willing and able to run. But most of the time I will be hiking. In fact, my average speed for the entire trip will likely hover somewhere between 3 and 3.5 miles per hour. Most hikers never realize that I am out trying to set a record. They just think that I am a day hiker or a really slow trail runner.

How are you feeling, now that the attempt is finally here?

EXCITED!!! I love the trail and I can't wait to be on it. Like I said earlier, I am tired of talking the talk. So this is a good point for me to sign off—and go and do my thing. I hope everyone gets some great hiking in this summer!

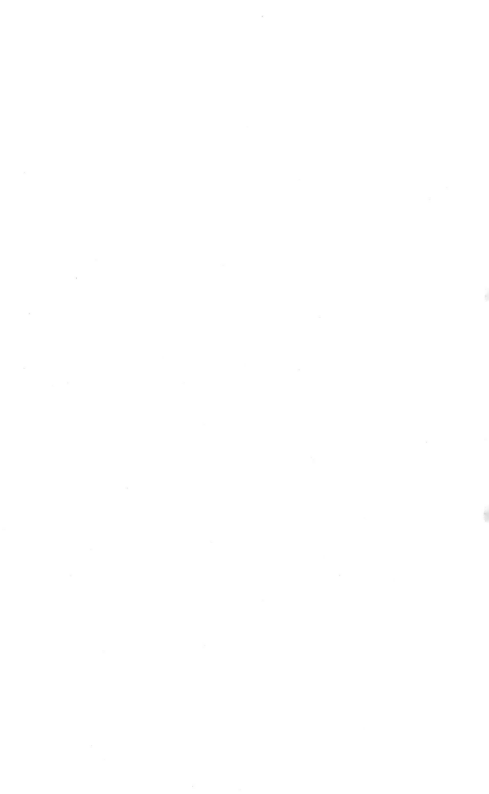

46 DAYS

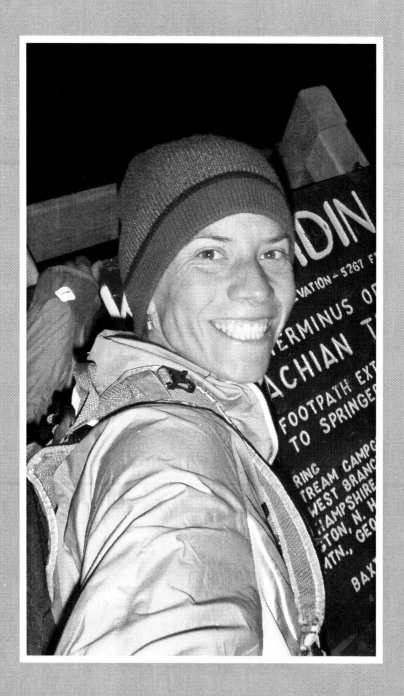

DAY 1
56 MILES

START TIME: 4:06 AM   ✦   END TIME: 9:15 PM

Jen shoved off from the base of Katahdin really early and touched the sign that marks the start of the trail at 4:06 AM. She was out of Baxter State Park (14+ miles from Katahdin's summit) by 8 AM and was able to hike quickly for the rest of the day because she's fresh, the weather's good, and the terrain's pretty easy—no mountains yet.

For every mile that Jen hikes in Maine, her support crew will have to drive about 3 miles to reach her. A lot of those miles are on dirt logging roads where we can't drive faster than 30 mph. Warren found out yesterday that a bridge was being rebuilt on one of the roads. It would have kept us from reaching her for re-supply early on Day 2, so we had to split up. Melissa and I took the three re-supplies this afternoon and Warren drove around to the other side of the bridge so he could re-supply her first thing in the morning. This is the kind of choreography that can make a difference on a hike like this and it's a LOT easier when you have a trail guru like Warren with you.

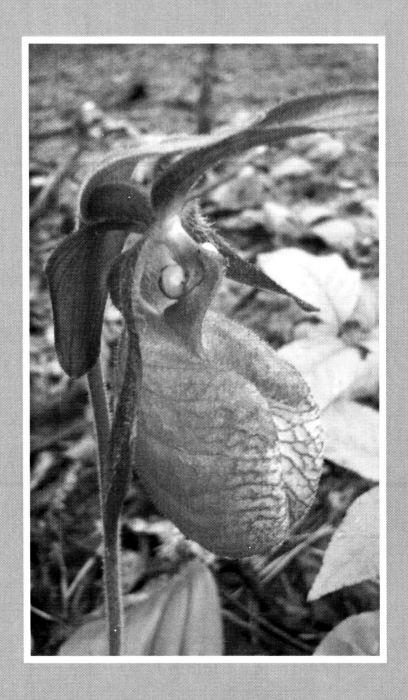

DAY 2

44 MILES

Jen got over her first major mountains today (besides Katahdin)—White Cap and Chairback—and made it through another big chunk of the 100 Mile Wilderness. She has TONS of black fly and mosquito bites on her scalp and behind her knees, but the rest of her body is holding up pretty well and she's in VERY good spirits. We brought her an enormous BBQ sandwich from Spring Creek BBQ in Monson and she scarfed it down. Our friend Melissa hiked in to give Jen some company during the mid-day stretch while I tried to help a dad and two sons from Freeport (home of L.L. Bean) find their wife/mom around Katahdin Iron Works. Two hours later they did reconnect, so that was a happy ending. Warren hiked in at dusk and helped Jen to get into camp safely. She tweaked her ankle right before bed, but we're hoping it won't prove to be a problem.

animal sightings: Melissa and I saw a moose this morning on our way to Katahdin Iron Works Road and Warren saw one while he was driving the other way around in his car. We saw an *enormous* snapping turtle, maybe 15 pounds, on our way in to the last rendezvous of the evening.

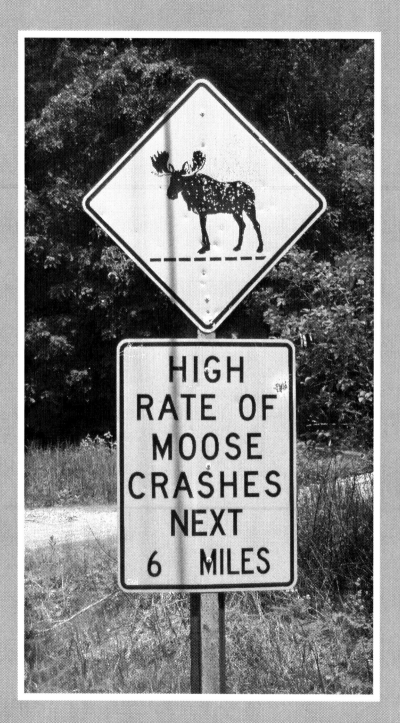

DAY 3
46 MILES

Jen had a great morning and covered the first 15 miles before 9 AM. We brought her chocolate donuts and coffee, which she ate while I put bug spray on her and filled her new socks with Gold Bond powder. At one point, she said, "This is the LIFE! Hiking the trail is worth it with this kind of treatment." Apparently she really likes having three people dote on her at each road crossing. I guess I wasn't enough last time she went after a record on the AT.

Melissa hiked with her for a mid-day stretch. I brought her a big sausage, onion, and pepper sandwich from Spring Creek in Monson, which she inhaled. I also brought her a whoopie pie, which is basically a big, soft homemade Oreo-type cookie that's popular up here in New England, but she hasn't eaten it yet. If she doesn't eat it soon, it's going to disappear into my belly.

She was hurting a little this afternoon—I guess hiking 125 miles in 2.5 days will eventually catch up to you—but she wanted to push on, and she made it to 5 miles outside of Caratunk by nightfall.

Melissa and I drank blueberry wheat beer and checked the internet at the Kennebec Brewery and Outfitters, and I spent some time sitting in a scalding hot tub. It was an awesome afternoon. Making some of these stops (Spring Creek BBQ, the hot tub, etc.) is like visiting old friends from the first trip.

Melissa and I saw a porcupine! It was AWESOME! Very quill-y. It was darker than I thought it'd be: black with yellow on the tips of the quills.

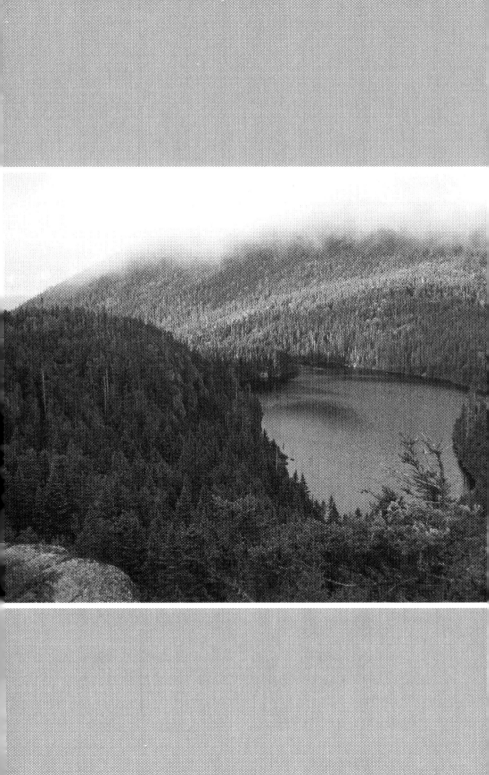

DAY 4
42 MILES

Another great day on the trail. Jen got to fulfill a dream of hers this morning: fording the Kennebec River. The Kennebec is the most legendary ford on the AT. Since 1985, outfitters in Caratunk have provided a canoe ferry twice a day so that hikers can avoid walking through the river, but Jen had her heart set on walking across. The water level was too high when we arrived at 6 AM (they raise and lower it at different times for the rafters upstream) so we went to an outfitter/lodge to soak in the hot tub, shower, and eat a big breakfast before heading back out at 7:45. The water level had gone down a foot or two to the point that Warren, who has forded the river two or three dozen times, felt comfortable about the two of them crossing it. So Warren led her across, dropped her off at the trail, and then forded back again. "Hardcore" is the best term I can think of to describe what they did. When Warren came back across, he howled, then bellowed, "I may have the face of a 61-year-old and the belly of a couch potato, but I've still got the legs of a WILD RIVER MAN!" Then he struck the Atlas pose and flexed his calves. It was awesome.

Jen's adrenaline was pumping after the river ford. She hiked strong in the late morning and early afternoon before reaching the Bigalow Mountains. Melissa hiked with her a few miles from there and then hiked in to her again as she came down the mountain last night. She had chili beef and mac with cheddar cheese and Fritos for dinner (thanks to Diamond Brand Outfitters in Asheville for the Mountain House meal!) and she did finally eat the whoopie pie, so no whoopie pie for me yet. Overall, it was another great day for the hiker princess.

animal sightings: I saw a red fox this morning while driving to the Kennebec, and the girls had two separate encounters with protective mommas. A momma deer stood her ground and snorted at Melissa in the early morning, and a momma grouse charged Jen on foot then dive-bombed her a few times in the late afternoon.

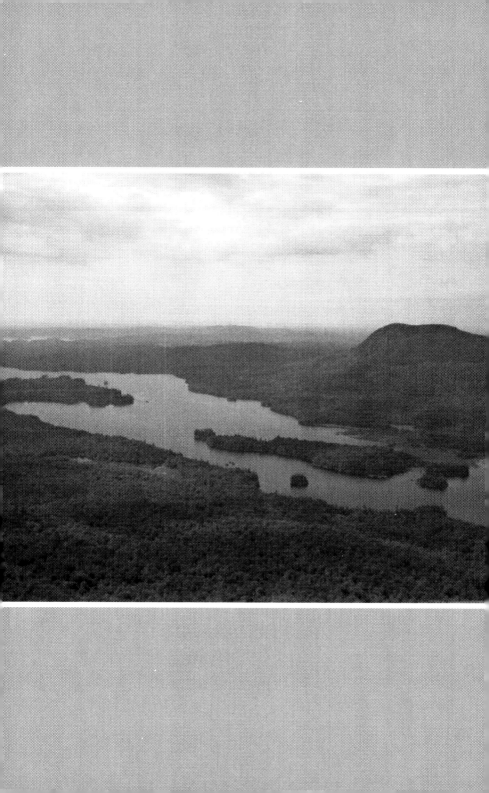

DAY 5
41 MILES

Today was pretty tough for Jen.

She wiped out coming down Crocker Mountain this morning and cut her knee up a little bit, then she fell a few minutes later when she was hiking with Melissa. She got to the first road crossing a few minutes late and was upset about the falls but in good spirits overall. While she was eating chocolate donuts and drinking hot tea, she said, "Maine's trying to EAT me!"

She was dragging a little the rest of the day because of the falls and the sleep deprivation since she only got 3-4 hours of sleep the first night, and 5-6 hours the other three, but she made it over Spaulding Mountain, and down to ME 4 (Rangeley) where she had pizza and Ben & Jerry's Peanut Butter Cup ice cream for dinner (she ate ALMOST the whole pint). Melissa hiked the last 8.5 miles with her and she hit the sack as soon as she got in, so she managed a solid 7 hours of sleep. Don't tell her I said this, but I think it was the first time I've ever heard her snore. Her left shin is bothering her, but we're hoping she'll put in another solid day tomorrow and make it to Grafton Notch.

animal sightings: Jen saw another moose yesterday—a mooseling—and I forgot to mention she had seen a moose the day before, in addition to the momma grouse. Loons serenaded us to sleep last night, and they sounded beautiful.

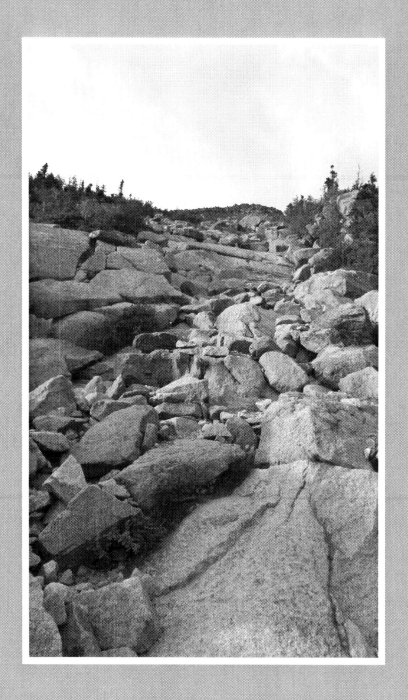

DAY 6
38 MILES

START TIME: 5:15 AM ✦ END TIME: 9:55 PM

Another grueling day. Jen slept an extra hour last night and was feeling much more rested when she woke up, but the shin splint in her left leg was bothering her all day. When I saw her in the late morning after she'd hiked 18 miles, she said, "It hurts on the uphills and the flats, but it's *excruciating* on the downhills." She hiked 10 miles with Melissa in the early afternoon and then another 10 with Warren into Grafton Notch. She got in later than expected last night and she was pretty drained emotionally and physically.

While she was icing down her shin and eating gobs of Moosetracks ice cream, she said this was her most painful injury ever, more painful than the badly sprained ankle on her 2008 AT hike, which was the size of a softball for 5-6 days, and the twisted knee on her 2007 Long Trail hike, when she walked 40+ miles through the pain for over two days. She's the toughest person I know and it's really hard to see her hurting so much—especially since I can't be out there on the trail with her—but Melissa has really stepped it up by hiking big miles with her. Warren continues to come through in a variety of ways, like finding roads and trails that no one knew existed, hiking in and out as much as possible, and giving lots of advice on how to handle the injury, so we keep fighting the good fight.

animal sightings: I saw the rump of a young black bear as it ran down a dirt road near Andover, Maine, in the mid-morning, and Jen saw another young moose and got charged a second time by another angry momma grouse.

DAY 7

31 MILES

START TIME: 6:10 AM   ✦   END TIME: 9:10 PM

Three big accomplishments today. First, Jen made it through the Mahoosuc Range—not the tallest, but probably the *toughest* mountains on the trail. Second, she made it out of Maine, which means no more black flies! But the biggest accomplishment was just getting out of bed this morning. Her shins had been KILLING her when she got to Grafton Notch last night. I was really thinking she might not hike anymore. This morning, she woke up at 4 and her shins still killed. Then she woke up at 5 and they were still intensely painful. But then she woke up at 6 and decided to try to walk around a bit with the hiking pole. She said her shins felt a little better, so she decided to "woman up" and keep going. She tackled Mahoosuc Notch, the craziest mile on the trail, where she had to walk on all fours through a one-mile boulder field, at around 10:45. After she made it through that, she kept going and got to Gentian Pond around 4:30. She hiked down the trail outside of Gorham around 8:50 and I got to walk with her on the dirt road then the asphalt for about ⅔ of a mile.

There's no telling how her shins will hold up on the rocky terrain of the Presidentials, which she'll enter tomorrow. It hurt her to road walk on the asphalt this evening so I'm guessing it'll be pretty painful to walk on the rocks, especially on the downhills. But she's going to keep soldiering on until she her body tells her to stop. In the meantime, she'll keep taking ibuprofen and icing her shins. Regardless, very few people have made it out of Maine in 7 days. I'm not a trail historian but my guess would be only two or three, if that. So that's something to be proud of.

food: She ate her usual, a banana and Clif Bar, for breakfast, a turkey, bacon, and avocado sandwich from Subway for a late afternoon lunch, and a Mountain House mac and cheese with chocolate milk for dinner. Her normal snacks include healthy stuff like Clif Bars, honey stingers, trail mix, mixed nuts, granola bars, healthier chips (tortilla chips and pretzels) and different kinds of cheese (mostly string cheese and hunks of cheddar cheese). The junk food includes candy bars, cookies, less healthy chips (Fritos, Combos, and Kettle Chips), marshmallows, donuts, brownies, gummies (especially Sour Patch Kids), and ice cream. Most of the time she drinks water, fruit juice mixed with water, or Gatorade. We don't keep track of her caloric intake, but ideally she'll be eating about 6,000 a day, or three times the normal amount for a woman. She tries to eat one snack every hour.

animal sightings: Warren, Melissa, and I had to take about a 75-mile detour today because a logging road had been closed on the Maine-New Hampshire border. When we were about to reach New Hampshire, a giant moose hopped a guard rail and started running diagonally down the road in front of Warren's car. Warren saw it in time and slammed on the brakes. There were some nice tire marks where he skidded to a stop. The moose didn't seem too concerned. He just kept loping across the road and onto the bank on the far side. Melissa had been wanting a close encounter with a moose, but I don't think she pictured it *that* way.

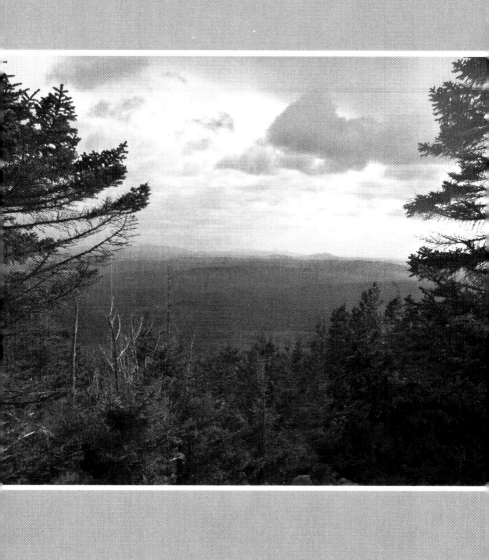

DAY 8
34 MILES

START TIME: 5:30 AM ✦ END TIME: 10:45 PM

Jen began the Presidentials today.

Melissa met her at Zeta Pass around noon, and we all met her at Pinkham Notch around 3:30. She asked me to bring her a crispy chicken sandwich and strawberry shake from McDonald's in Gorham. I guess hiking's a little like being pregnant. I never know what Jen's going to be craving.

It was cloudy most of the day. We were hoping the rain would hold off long enough for Jen to make it to the summit of Mt. Washington then on to the hut, but the rain and fog came in and she didn't get quite get that far. She and Warren had to be resourceful about finding shelter, but in general they stayed warm and dry.

By my very rough calculations, Jen climbed about 13,700 feet (almost ½ of Everest) today and descended 5700 feet, after averaging 42 miles a day for a full week, over some of the toughest terrain of the AT, with hurting shins. My wife is a BEAST! But then again, it could all end tomorrow with a bad fall or if the shin splints get worse instead of better.

So far, Jen has been able to neutralize the pain by taping them while she walks, icing them while she's sitting, taking LOTS of anti-inflammatories, and stretching them gently. We got great treatment advice from Jen's college roommate, Emily, who is a physical trainer. She has been very helpful.

As Winston Churchill said, "When you're going through hell, keep going." We're hoping to get through the Whites in one piece in another day and a half.

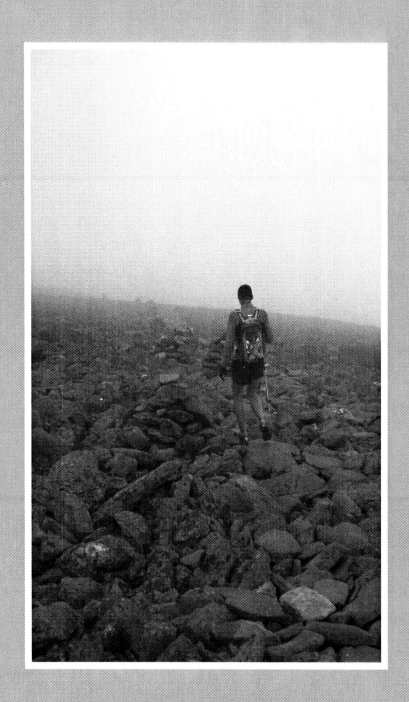

DAY 9
30 MILES

START TIME: 5:30 AM   ✦   END TIME: 8:30 PM

Jen had a rainy, messy day in the White Mountains of New Hampshire, the most rugged and exposed range in the eastern United States. She and Warren stopped for a quick coffee at Lakes of the Clouds Hut, so that Jen could warm up, then they went their separate ways: Warren back to his car at Pinkham Notch and Jen toward ours at Crawford Notch. Unfortunately, she hiked two or three miles on the wrong trail before realizing her mistake and turning around. The AT isn't marked well in the Whites, and it's marked even less well for southbounders than north-bounders, since so few people thru-hike that way. She got to Crawford Notch a couple hours late and was frustrated about the wrong turn. Fortunately, after we cranked Mumford & Sons and peeled off her wet clothes, she was upbeat again. After she left the car around 2 PM, Melissa, Warren, and I drove around to the Gale River trailhead where Melissa hiked up 3.5 miles to meet Jen and camp for the night. If all goes well, Jen will get out of the Whites (and maybe the crummy weather) tomorrow night.

injury report: We were worried that the mega-downhill from Mt. Washington would do a number on her shins but so far the tape, ibuprofen, and walking with a pole have been working. She has also started wearing compression socks. They are called Salomon EXO calves, and they help retain energy in her legs and offer support. She says she doesn't need to ice her shins because the cold rain is just as effective. I'm not sure I buy that, but as long as her legs aren't bothering her, she can do whatever she wants. **She is, after all, hiking 40+ miles a day.**

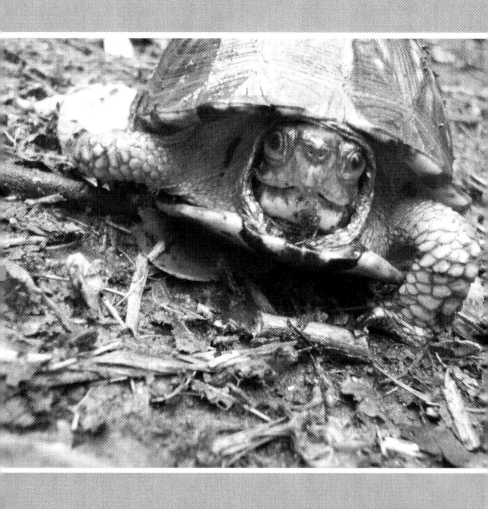

DAY 10

38 MILES

START TIME: 4:45 AM ✦ END TIME: 9:15 PM

Well, it was an incredibly challenging day with more nasty weather, but we are officially out of the Whites! Jen camped with Melissa last night at the Gale River trail junction. Melissa said she didn't get much sleep because of two things: the driving wind and Jen's snoring. (In her defense, Jen has never snored before. I'm sure she's doing it because she's congested from all the hiking.) Anyway, Warren slept at the Gale River trailhead and I slept down in Franconia Notch, where Jen arrived around 10:30 this morning.

Today proved more difficult, weather-wise, than either of the two previous days. She had to walk through sleet and 25-30 mph winds on Franconia Ridge, an exposed ridgeline, for several miles before getting below the tree line. When she got to the tent, she climbed in a sleeping bag to warm up, then she inhaled the two sausage McMuffins and coffee that Warren brought her from the McDonald's in Lincoln. After that she was ready to go again.

She climbed North and South Kinsman Mountains in the early afternoon and came flying into Kinsman Notch around 4:45. When she hit the parking lot, she pumped her fist and yelled "Come on!" like she'd just won a big point in a tennis match. She was only in the car for 10 minutes or so before she headed back out to climb Moosilauke, the last big mountain in the Whites. Warren, Melissa, and I drove into Warren, NH, where we got some pizza for Jen and took fun photos of Warren eating hot dogs in front of the sign at the Warren Convenience Store.

We reached Glencliff at about 7 PM and Melissa hiked toward Moosilauke to make sure Jen got down all right. I re-heated her pizza on the stove then walked in for about 10 minutes, and got to deliver the line I came up with earlier: "Did someone order a plain cheese pizza?" It was hysterical. At least to me.

I got to road walk with Jen for about 1/3 of a mile before she and Melissa hiked the last mile or so through the woods. Overall, it was a GREAT day. The weather conditions were certainly not ideal, but we made it out of the Whites without any serious problems, and now Jen has just 43 more miles til she's in Vermont. We're thrilled and awed with what the little hiker princess has been able to do so far.

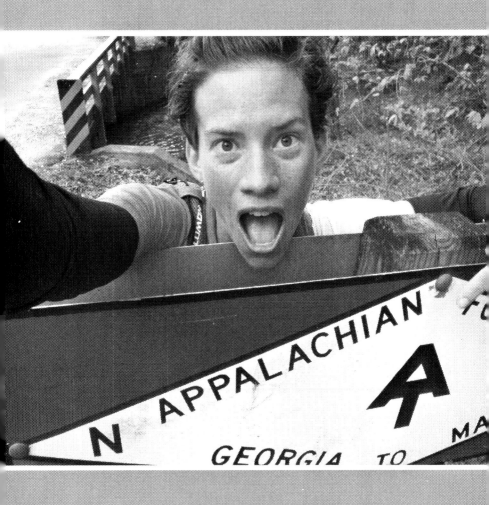

DAY 11

43 MILES

START TIME: 4:30 AM ✦ END TIME: 10:15 PM

We made it to Hanover! Jen was really hurting this morning. Warren said she was running on adrenaline when she was above tree line in the Whites, and now that that's over, she's going to have to settle down into a routine with less excitement but no less work.

There were low clouds and fog again all day today, but it only rained for about half an hour right after dark. Jen arrived at the third road crossing at about 2 o'clock and was frustrated that she didn't have more energy, but she really picked it up this afternoon and cranked out the last 19 miles at a much faster pace than the first 24.

A big part of that was that Melissa hiked with her for the last *18 miles* of the day. It's been awesome how Melissa has stepped up since Jen's shin splints started hurting. Melissa primarily came along to shoot photos and video footage, and maybe hike a little bit when she had time, but those priorities have definitely changed in the last week or so. She's been hiking big chunks of the trail with Jen, keeping her company and making sure she doesn't have to take extra steps at ambiguous trail junctions.

Another big encouragement the second half of the day was when Jen's friend J ("Mooch" to those of you who've read Jen's memoir about her first thru-hike, *Becoming Odyssa*) drove down from St. Johnsbury, Vermont, to keep Jen and Melissa company for the last two or three miles and help set up camp.

Jen continues to impress us with her perseverance. In spite

of the shin splints, sleep deprivation (she's used to getting 9 hours and she's been getting 6), and continued dreary weather, she's maintaining a very strong pace and an upbeat attitude.

food: I got to eat an enormous bacon cheeseburger and fries from Murphy's in Hanover. We brought Jen a chicken burrito from Boloco for lunch and chicken pad thai and red curry with steak from Mai Thai for dinner. She's eating well and seems to be maintaining her weight better than last time, when she lost 15 pounds in the first four weeks.

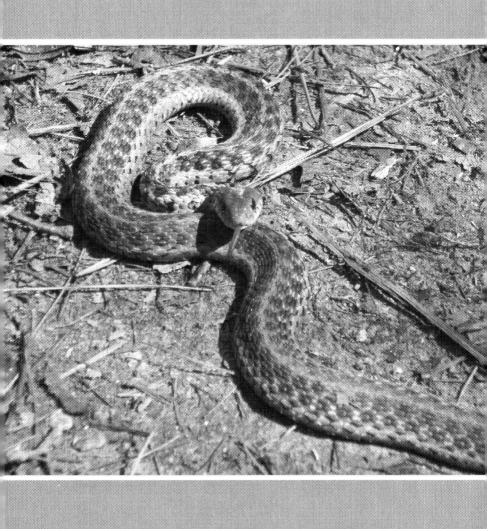

DAY 12
36 MILES

This was definitely Jen's toughest day, physically and emotionally. She slept in a bit this morning, then did a couple miles of road walking through Hanover and Norwich, Vermont, which really hurt her shins. Later in the morning, she had another road walk—this time downhill—and she was in even more pain. She got through all of that and was making good time into the early evening.

Around 6 PM, Melissa and I were heading back to the trail from the Long Trail Brewery when we got a call from Jen saying she'd had diarrhea all afternoon. It's possible she got it from the kielbasa sausage and pint of Ben & Jerry's "Everything but the . . ." ice cream she had for lunch, but her stomach had been bothering her before that, just not so intensely.

Anyway, she said she was really struggling and that she didn't think she could make it to Hwy 4 in Killington (which would have been a 46-mile day) and that we should plan on camping at the River Road about 6 miles short of that. When we got to that road crossing at around 7, Melissa started hiking in. Around 8:15, I got a call from Jen saying she'd run into Adam and Kadrah Cassidy, a young couple from Elkins, West Virginia. Adam ran the Mountain Masochist last fall and introduced himself to us after the race and told Jen he was going to try to run the AT this summer. That was the last we saw or heard from him until yesterday when Jen stumbled out of the backwoods of Vermont onto a random dirt road and heard Adam yell her name. Jen told me later that when she saw

them, she was so zapped and depleted from her stomach issues
that she wouldn't have gotten to our road crossing before mid-
night without their help, and that she definitely would have
quit the record attempt.

From there, Kadrah drove Jen to Gifford Woods State Park
where Warren and I met them. Jen took a shower, then we
headed out the Stony Brook Road to camp. Melissa called me
and was concerned that she hadn't run into Jen and that it was
starting to rain and it was getting dark and the trails were getting more treacherous. I told her what had happened and that
she shouldn't worry about Jen but she should keep hiking and
reach the road to meet Adam.

We are Christians and have asked for prayers from friends
and family throughout this adventure—not prayers for success, but prayers for safety. Some people would say Jen just
happened to run into this couple by coincidence, but we believe
in a God who answers prayers and who performs miracles. We
believe that God provided for Jen, and Adam and Kadrah felt
the same way.

This divine encounter and the fact that Jen's flashlight went
out right after she touched the sign on top of Mt. Washington
are proof to us that God has answered our prayers and that he
has kept her safe and healthy so far.

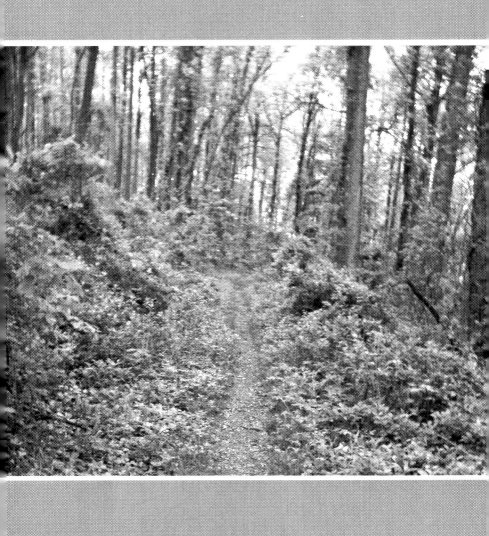

DAY 13
42.5 MILES

START TIME: 5:30 AM   ✦   END TIME: 10:20 PM

Jen's stomach problems continued this morning. It took her 5.5 hours to hike the first 10.5 miles. She had to use the bathroom every 20 minutes, and she was totally depleted. We had a talk at the road crossing and decided she should press on through the discomfort. I had no idea what to expect at the next road crossing. I thought it might take her forever to make the 12 miles or that we might even have to go in and get her. To our surprise, though, she came chugging toward the road around 3:30. She thanked me for encouraging her to keep hiking, ate a Whopper, and kept plugging right along to the next road crossing where she ate a big ham, turkey, and cheese sandwich.

She covered 32 miles over the last 10.5 hours of the day, which is substantially faster than her pace has been up to this point. Her shins weren't bothering her as much, she was upbeat in general, but especially happy that her stomach was feeling better and that we were filling it with burgers, pepperoni pizza, OJ, and whatever else she was willing to eat. The first two weeks have really been a roller coaster ride emotionally and physically. We're hoping that the health issues are behind us and that Jen can settle into some sort of rhythm as we near the kinder, gentler mid-Atlantic states.

gear: Some people have been asking about Jen's gear. Salomon has provided her with new trail shoes called the Synapse. She LOVES them, and they're very stylish, too—light blue with peachy soles. I think they'll be out later this year. All of her clothes are Salomon. We got Clif Bars and Honey Stingers from our AWESOME local outdoor store, Diamond Brand Outfitters, and we're still using the lightweight Snow Peak stove and Western Mountaineering 40-degree down sleeping bags they gave us from Jen's last record-attempt hike. That has all held up well the past few summers of hiking in Colorado and Europe. Diamond Brand has a website so you can buy stuff online if you don't live in western North Carolina.

We got hiking poles and a great lightweight tent from Easton Mountain Products called the Kilo. If my memory serves me correctly from secondary school science classes, I'm guessing it weighs 2.2 pounds. Pretty darn light and very comfortable for two people. Also easy to put up.

We're sleeping on these snazzy new pads from Klymit called Inertia X-Frames. I've mentioned twice how much Jen is snoring so you know how comfortable those are. We also have this fantastic all-natural bug spray 45 N, 63 W. I was skeptical that all-natural bug spray would work as well as DEET, but it has worked just as well if not better. So that's the scoop on gear.

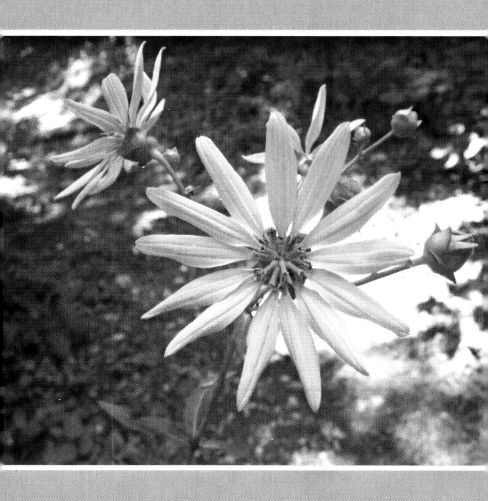

DAY 14

43.5 MILES

START TIME: 5:10 AM   ✦   END TIME: 9:30 PM

Jen had a great day. She got an early start from Danby-Landgrove Road and reached Mad Tom Notch around 9:45. She made good time over Bromley Mountain and reached VT 11/30 around lunchtime where we all ran into the president of the Green Mountain Club. She was out there painting blazes with another volunteer, and she and Jen had a nice chat about the Long Trail while Jen ate lunch. She's been wanting to eat healthier, heartier meals recently so I've been making things like deli sandwiches and chicken salad wraps. They don't have as many calories, but I think Jen's sick of all the junk food.

We made a logistical error this afternoon and tried to make it up Stratton Mountain two different ways to cut Jen's 17.5-mile stretch into 11.2- and 6.3-mile stretches. The gazetteers usually show where there are gates, but it didn't show them this time so we hit two dead ends. It ended up being a minor mistake though, because we reached Jen on her cell phone and she had enough food and clothes and was making good time. Warren highlighted good road crossings for us in the databook and gazetteer before he left two days ago, and the road we tried wasn't one of them. The moral of this story is always listen to the Trail Yoda.

Jen reached Stratton-Arlington Road around 5:30, and Forest Road 71 by 6:10, where she and Melissa loaded up their packs. Melissa carried most of the camping gear so Jen's pack could be as light as possible, and they hiked a little further and camped just past Kid Gore Shelter. They'd planned to go a bit further than that, but it started raining and they were climbing up a steep ascent. It turned out to be a good decision because a thunderstorm rolled in just a few minutes later.

Jen's been trying to air out her shins because the tape has given them a rash or infection or something. The shin splints themselves seem to be doing better. We keep icing them and she keeps taking ibuprofen and elevating them when she takes breaks.

Aside from the nighttime thunderstorm, it hasn't rained on us much, but the trail conditions have still been messy because there's been a lot of rain in Vermont the past few weeks. Jen loves heat and sunshine, so we're hoping things will dry out a bit in Massachusetts.

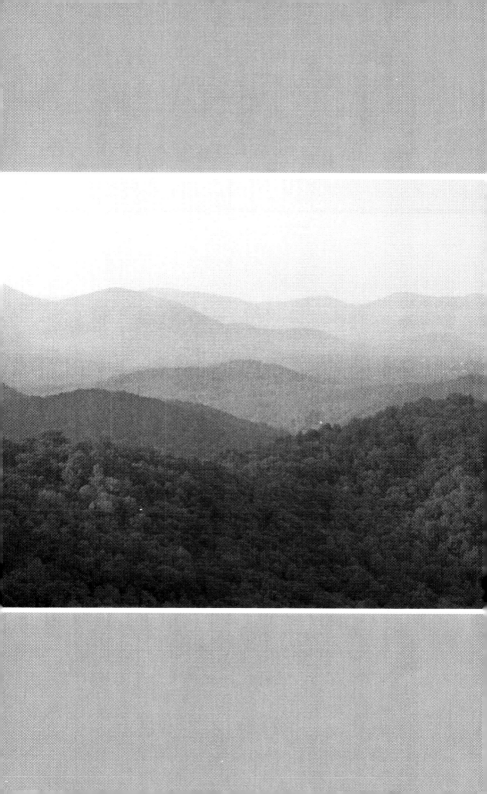

DAY 15
47.3 MILES

START TIME: 5:00 AM   ✦   END TIME: 10:10 PM

Jen hiked really strong today. Melissa camped out with Jen last night. When they woke up, Jen put in 14 miles down to VT 9 and got to the road crossing about 10 AM. Melissa packed up the tent and gear and made it out about an hour later. I had enough time in between to run into Bennington and pick up some shoes from home that the best neighbors in the world, Frank and Lauren, mailed to us.

Jen reached County Road (4 miles north of the Vermont-Massachusetts border) in the early afternoon and crossed into Massachusetts around 3 PM. We got to road-walk together through North Adams and then hike another short, flat stretch on the way up Mt. Graylock. Aside from sleeping, time together for us has been rare, so it was great to have an extra 30-40 minutes to catch up.

Jen summited Graylock (the tallest mountain in Massachusetts) a little after 7 pm as the clouds were rolling in and a light rain was starting to fall. Melissa and I drove around to Cheshire and Melissa hiked in from Outlook Avenue. They reached Outlook Avenue just before 9:30 and MA Highway 8 about 15 minutes later. I got to walk the last half-mile into town with Jen. It was her biggest mileage day since Day 1. Something to be very proud of.

I convinced a family near the trail to let Jen use their outdoor shower, so she was able to clean off all the cuts on her leg. (One woman at Clarendon Gorge in Vermont had commented on how bruised and battered Jen's legs were and gave me a nasty look. I'm pretty sure she thought I was abusing her.) Then we crashed at St. Mary of the Assumption Catholic Church. Thanks to Father David and the parishioners for their kindness and hospitality!

Right now, Jen's in good shape physically. The shin splints aren't hurting as much, none of the cuts are infected, and we're hoping the stomach problems won't come back.

As a sidebar, some of you know that when Jen set the record in 2008, I referred to myself as her sherpa. About a week ago, I decided to call this year's group—Melissa, Warren, Horton, Steve Feller, myself, and the others who have been enlisted to offer support along the way—the Pit Crew. You know, because we have to get Jen in and out as quickly as possible at the road crossings (like NASCAR), and because we don't get to shower very often so our armpits smell awful.

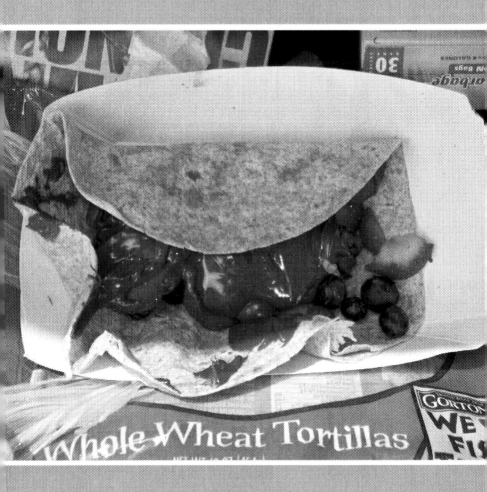

DAY 16
48.7 MILES

START TIME: 5:00 AM   ✦   END TIME: 9:45 PM

Jen's relatively healthy and the trail's less demanding, and both of these things are leading to bigger miles. She left Cheshire at the crack of dawn and made it to Gulf Road outside of Dalton, Massachusetts, by 7:30. I got to road walk with her for about a mile. It was nice to have that extra time to catch up.

After the pit stop, Melissa and I got pancakes and omelets at a little diner, then went grocery shopping for deli meats and smoothies. I found a chocolate smoothie with LOTS of protein and Jen chugged an entire 32-ounce bottle yesterday (760 calories). When she's doing these endurance hikes, she gets tired of chewing so she was happy I found the smoothies.

Melissa and I drove around to Washington Mountain Road, where I hiked with Jen for a flat ½-mile stretch. Right after that, we ran into a guy named Tim Meadows who's from Hendersonville, North Carolina, of all places (Jen's home town), and who's finishing up a section hike after 35 years. Thumbs up for that!

Melissa and I went with Tim to a blueberry farm just down the road where a couple named the Wileys provide homemade cookies and sodas to thru-hikers. We chatted with all of them for a bit then headed out.

Jen reached US 20 outside of Lee by mid-afternoon. Melissa hiked an 8-mile stretch with her while I went into Great Barrington to pick up some uber-lightweight carbon hiking poles from Easton Mountain Products. Jen had been craving protein earlier so I picked up an Angus burger and fries from

McDonald's then headed out to Tyringham to meet up with her and Melissa.

She hiked another 12 miles from there down to Mass 23 outside of Great Barrington. Melissa hiked in from Blue Hill Road near Mass 23 while I made their dinners. (Jen's was an 840-calorie Chicken and Rice from Mountain House.)

Jen's still taking ibuprofen and elevating her feet at road crossings, and we ice her shins when we can, but she's feeling as healthy right now as she has since we started this thing 16 days ago. We really appreciate all the encouraging e-mails and phone calls we've received from everyone.

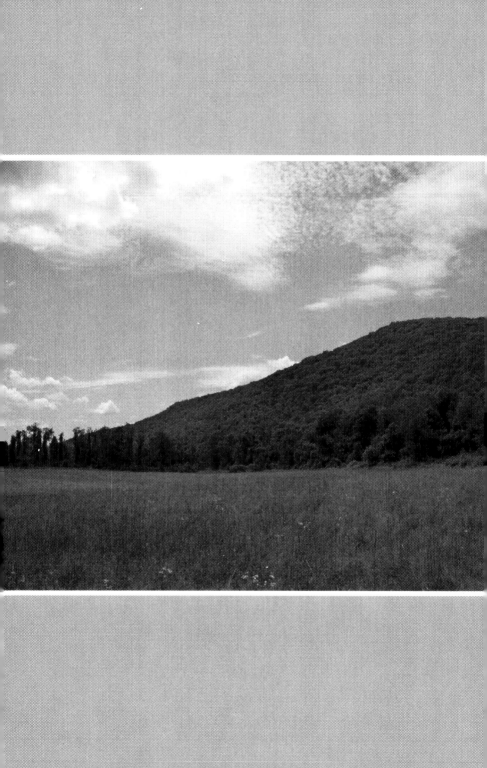

DAY 17

48.3 MILES

START TIME: 5:05 AM   ✦   END TIME: 9:20 PM

Jen put in another very strong day. She reached US 7 outside of Sheffield, Massachusetts, by about 7:30 AM. Melissa and I got bagels and coffee at the Great Barrington Bagel Company. We kind of stumbled onto it without realizing how good it was. It was packed for the 4th of July weekend.

Jen hiked the next 4.5 miles to Jug End Road so fast that she was about 50 yards from the road as we pulled up. From there she had a big 17-mile stretch to Salisbury. She was feeling good and said she didn't need Melissa to hike in so we did some laundry in Lakeville and checked e-mail at the Scoville Memorial Library, the first public library in the United States. It was beautiful. The outside looked like an old stone church.

After four hours or so, we drove to the trail crossing north of Salisbury and waited for Jen. She got there about 3 o'clock, and I got to walk with her on a short, flat stretch of trail and road.

When she left, Melissa and I swung by Mizza's Pizza in Lakeville. I got a pepperoni and meatball calzone for Jen and me to split, and Melissa got spaghetti and meatballs. We each had a Long Trail Ale and then the owner offered us another, I think because he thought we were waiting for our to-go order. Anyway, it was generous of him.

Jen reached the Iron Bridge near Falls Village around 5:30. She scarfed down her calzone and then kept walking. Our buddy Steve Feller met us about 45 minutes later and hiked the last 7 miles or so with Jen into West Cornwall Road. She stopped a little early today because she'd done a great job, she wanted to shower, and because she'd kind of tweaked her shin earlier in the day and she didn't want to push it.

Melissa went back to Steve's house for the night (he lives in Mahopac, New York) and I drove Jen down to the Housatonic Meadows State Park for a shower. She ate Melissa's leftover spaghetti and meatballs on the way. She was pretty zonked when we got back to the tent, but since she finished early, she also got to bed earlier.

We're glad to have Steve with us for a few days. He's a strong runner and hiker and will be able to pace Jen and push her—not literally, of course—when she needs it.

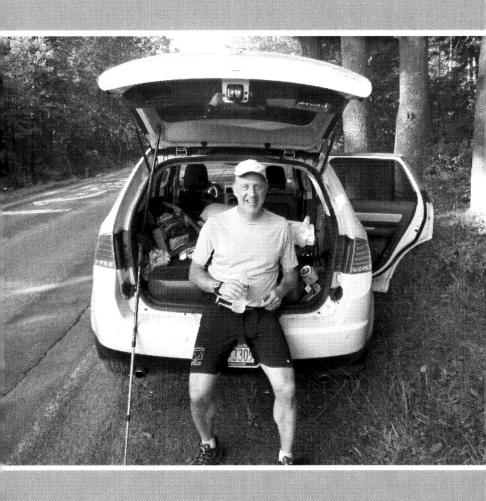

DAY 18
49 MILES

Jen had another strong day with big miles. It took her about 2 hours to hike the first 5-mile stretch. She was a little disappointed with that pace, but the rest of the day she hiked fast. So fast that our friend Steve Feller, an accomplished trail runner who's completed an Ironman triathlon and numerous 100-mile races, hiked with her for about 10 miles then had to take a break until it got dark because, as he said, "She's running me into the ground." And so fast that later in the day, Melissa and I missed her at a road crossing.

It turned out all right, but I was furious with myself at the time. We had reached NY 55 outside of Poughquag around 6:30 PM. Jen had a 7.6 mile stretch, and she'd left the previous road (NY 22) at 5:35. NY 55 is a major highway so we couldn't set up on the side of the road like we usually do. We had to park in a lot about 50 yards down the road in the woods. But there was a short side trail that led to the AT.

I figured Melissa and I could sit in the car until 7:35 because Jen hasn't been running and I didn't think she could average 3.5 mph walking. But apparently she can. We took the chairs, drinks, and snacks and got to the trail junction a few minutes late. We waited for a while then I decided to walk in because the section was relatively flat. After 15-20 minutes I didn't see her so I was assuming she was just hiking slow. I was getting a little worried after hiking in almost a mile.

Then around 8:05, I got a call from a 610 number. I didn't recognize the number, but we've had enough incidents like this over the years that I know to answer the phone because it could be Jen calling. And it was. She'd passed the trail junction a couple of minutes before we got there. She still had 30 minutes or so of daylight so she wanted to hike on to the next road crossing at Depot Hill Road and wait for us there. We figured she and Melissa could hike the last 5 miles with their headlamps. That is, of course, assuming we could find her.

We had great road maps for Maine, New Hampshire, Vermont, and Massachusetts, but for some reason, you can't find detailed maps of Connecticut and New York in the average gas station. It's probably because—unlike Jen and me—most people live in the 21st century and have moved on to things like GPS, iPods, and 4G cell phones.

We do have an iPad for the summer, but we couldn't pick up a signal so I just decided to start driving in the direction I thought the trail would be. I saw train tracks and figured Depot Hill Road might be near those, but the road we were on started winding away from the tracks. Eventually it deadended into a larger road and we saw a pizza place in a shopping center a couple hundred yards away. I ran in there and asked if anyone knew where Depot Hill Road was. One of the guys in the back came out and was able to tell me where to go. It took another 5 or 10 minutes for us to find her, but we did. She'd been waiting, she said, for about 20 minutes. She wasn't upset or frustrated, but she did say she could picture me having a few choice words for myself on the drive over. And she was right.

When Jen realized around 8 o'clock that we'd missed the re-supply and that it was getting dark, she didn't want to stop but she knew she had to find someone with a phone. She kept hiking and didn't see anyone, but then she smelled someone. What she really smelled was bug spray. She started looking around and eventually saw a couple camping nearby and asked to use their cell phone. They were kind and helpful and let her use the phone, then offered her water and snacks if she needed them. And an hour or two later, they called me to make sure she was OK.

Anyway, at the Depot Hill Road crossing, Melissa hiked in with Jen, I drove around to set up the tent, and Steve met us at NY 52 with an enormous New York-style pizza. He said it wasn't very good but we all loved it because we were hungry and happy that everything had worked out and that Jen had hiked 49 miles. So it was just another exciting day on the Appalachian Trail for Jen and her Pit Crew.

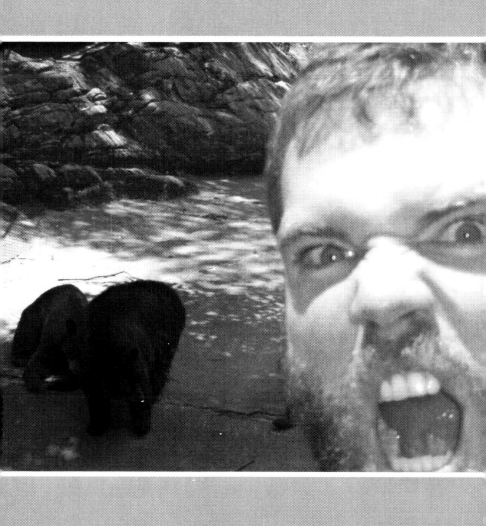

DAY 19
49 MILES

START TIME: 5:06 AM ✦ END TIME: 9:40 PM

Jen reached RPH Shelter a little before 7 AM and Canopus Lake by a little after 9. The next stretch was 12.1 miles and while she hiked it, Melissa, Steve, and I went back to Steve's house to do laundry, take care of trash and recycling, shower, watch the men's Wimbledon finals, and—wait for it—sit in the hot tub. That's right. While Jen was trudging through the mud and drizzling rain all morning, we were lounging in a hot tub and listening to music.

In addition to watching Djokavic beat Nadal and getting blasted by the super-strong jets in the hot tub, Steve's wife Mary Ellen made us the best chicken burgers in the world and we loaded them up with red onions, spinach, and avocado. She made a couple for Jen to eat on the trail and she also whipped up a fruit smoothie before we left. We were only at the Fellers' place for a couple hours, but it was easily the most relaxing and rejuvenating 2-hour stretch of the trail. Of course, I would have loved for Jen to have been there, but she was taking care of business.

She reached NY 9 around 1 PM and we walked across the Hudson River Bridge and through the Bear Mountain Zoo together before she and Steve headed up Bear Mountain to the Perkins Tower. Melissa hiked down with her to Seven Lakes Road and then Steve hiked the final 5.1 miles to Arden Valley Road. It rained most of the day, but Jen maintained a solid pace and avoided any major falls in the slippery conditions. Thanks for all the encouraging messages and the continued thoughts and prayers.

food: Jen's been drinking a lot of chocolate milk recently. She's also been eating a lot of whole milk yogurt and Greek yogurt with honey. She's been asking for more hand-held snacks (granola bars, pop tarts, candy bars, cookies, etc.) and less potato chips, trail mix, and other snacks that come in little pieces because the hand-held snacks let her focus more on the terrain and less on eating. She has been drinking Pepsi Throwback because it uses real sugar instead of high fructose corn syrup.

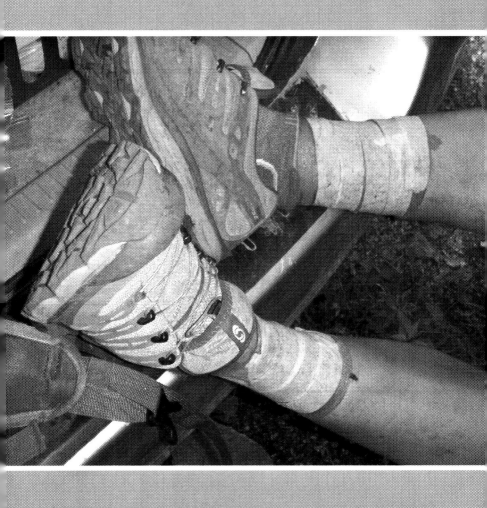

DAY 20
45 MILES

START TIME: 5:05 AM ✦ END TIME: 9:10 PM

Before I tell you about the day, I have to tell you about what happened in the middle of the night. At about 2 AM, I woke up to Jen pawing at the side of our tent and saying, "I have to get on the trail . . . I need to get on the trail!" She wasn't even awake. She was just sleep-talking and, I guess, trying to sleep-hike. I woke her up and she said, "Where are we?" I told her we were in the tent and that it was the middle of the night and she went back to sleep. Then we laughed about it in the morning.

As for Day 20, for the first time during the trip, the weather has been exactly how Jen wants it: hot and sunny. I met her after her first 9 miles at Lakes Road then the rest of the crew (Steve and Melissa, who have slept at Steve's place the past three nights) met us at NY 17A between Bellvale and Glenwood Lake. She bounced back and forth along the New York/New Jersey line for the entire day and there were tons of road crossings, so we probably got to see her 7 or 8 times. On the shortest of those stretches (2-3 miles), she doesn't carry anything. Not even water. On the longer ones, she sometimes carries her small daypack, and other times our buddy Steve carries a water bottle and snacks for her.

Steve's been powering out 15-20 miles every day, setting a torrid pace, and giving me "10-minute warning" phone calls when they near the road crossings. I love that because it gives me peace of mind and lets me know when to get ready for their arrival.

Mel night-hiked with Jen on the final stretch between Unionville and NJ 519 and they got in around 9 o'clock. Jen was feeling a little sluggish after the past week of averaging over 48 miles a day so she decided to stop an hour early and get an extra hour of sleep.

one other funny story: Jen's still taping her shins to make sure they're healthy for the rock fields of Pennsylvania. I asked her if the tape was irritating her skin or anything and she said, "No. I kind of like it now. It makes me feel like Zenyatta." If you don't know who Zenyatta is, look her up. It's a pretty fitting metaphor.

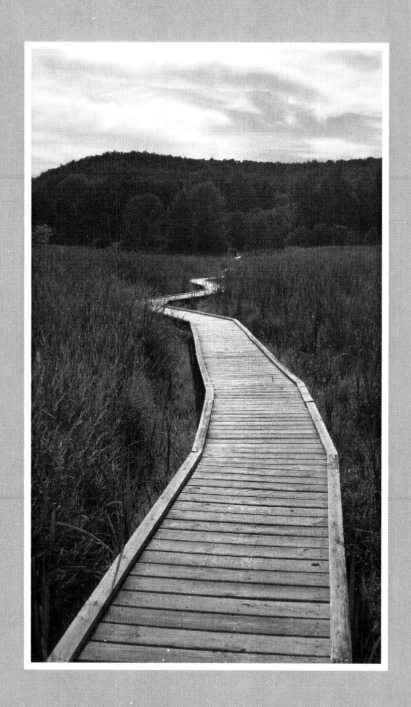

DAY 21

52.7 MILES

STAR TIME: 5:06 AM ✦ END TIME: 10:10 PM

This was Jen's biggest day on the trail, mileage-wise, since she put up 56 the first day. She woke up and left County Road 519 and hiked 11.9 miles to Sunrise Mountain. If you've read Jen's book, you know that this is where she came across the suicide victim. When Jen hiked in 2008, she wanted to stop at the Pavilion on top of the mountain (where she found the body) and pray. I assumed she'd want to do the same thing this time, but she had assumed that we would meet at the parking lot of the pavilion and not the pavilion itself. She was pretty shaken when she reached the top because she had wanted to prepare mentally in the parking lot and hadn't had a chance to do that since all the food, drinks, and supplies were with us at the pavilion. It was the sort of simple misunderstanding that happens when one person is hiking 45-50 miles a day and the other is trying to intuit things to make life easier.

I thought it might ruin Jen's mood for the rest of the day, but she was in a much better place at the next road crossing. She and Steve pounded out fast miles throughout the day. So fast, in fact, that she reached Delaware Water Gap a good hour and a half early. She decided to keep hiking, so she and Melissa, grabbed a couple slices of pepperoni pizza each and hiked another 7 miles to PA 191. While they were hiking, I was able to take a shower at the Presbyterian Church of the Mountain. I was also able to grab a homemade strawberry rhubarb pie from the pie shop in Delaware Water Gap (which is a town, not a river) and a second pepperoni pizza for Jen's and Mel's second dinner of the evening.

animal sightings: I haven't mentioned any animal sightings recently but that doesn't mean we're not having them. Jen's seen at least seven or eight bears in the past few days, the most recent being a big momma bear that was really close to the trail today. Jen saw her and walked right on past, and the bear just looked up for a second and went right on eating.

Mel heard a momma bear and her cubs near our campsite last night, and the girls both saw a porcupine. I read somewhere that New Jersey has more bears per square mile than any other state east of the Mississippi, and based the number of bear encounters we had in our two days in the state, I would say that's accurate.

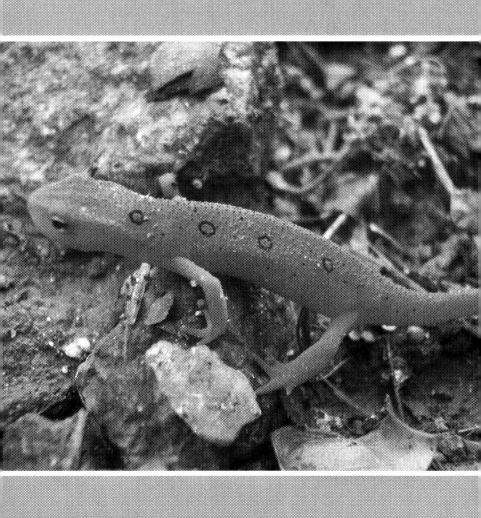

DAY 22
48 MILES

There were a lot of transitions today. Melissa's husband Ryan picked her up so she could photograph a friend's wedding in West Virginia. Steve drove home to New York to rest up before coming back out for the weekend. Jen's friend and publisher Eric Kampmann stopped by on his way from Virginia (where he was finishing a section hike) to his home in Connecticut. And we had two new members join the Pit Crew. Jim Eagleton (aka, "Rambler"), a thru-hiker Jen met in the Bigelows on Day 4, offered his services after he finished the trail. He lives north of Philadelphia, about an hour from where we are right now, so we recruited him and his friend Marnix (aka, "Dutch"), another thru-hiker from the Netherlands, to spend a couple of days with us at least until Steve gets back.

So there was all that transition, but all things considered it was another great day. Jen reached Wind Gap around 8 AM. Steve hiked in from Smith Gap to meet her, and he hiked in again at Little Gap and Lehigh Gap near Palmerton. Melissa hiked in with Steve at Little Gap, and then they both hit the road from Palmerton around 3:30 PM.

Rambler and Dutch met us at Lehigh Gap and after Jen headed out, the three of us met Eric in Slatington. We all drove up to Bake Oven Knob Road where Eric and Jen caught up for a few minutes. After that, Jen and I got to hike a mile-long flat stretch together.

Eric left from Bake Oven Knob Road, and Rambler, Dutch, and I drove around to Blue Mountain Summit, then on to Fort

Franklin Road where they hiked an extra three miles with Jen before setting up camp at dark.

The weather was great all day—hot and sunny—and the rocks haven't seemed to bother Jen too much yet. She brought a couple pairs of stiffer-soled XT Wing shoes for the rocky terrain in Pennsylvania. She wore them for the first 8 miles today, but then switched back to her faithful Synapses.

Since we've had so many transitions today and since we're just about at the halfway point, I want to take a minute to thank everyone who has helped out on the trail so far: Warren, Melissa, Steve, his wife Mary Ellen, Adam and Kadrah, Rambler and Dutch, Horton, and Eric. In some way or another, these people have put Jen's needs (and mine, too) above their own. They've sacrificed their own comfort for ours, and they've given their time and energy without asking for anything in return. There is absolutely no way we could have made it this far without you. So thanks.

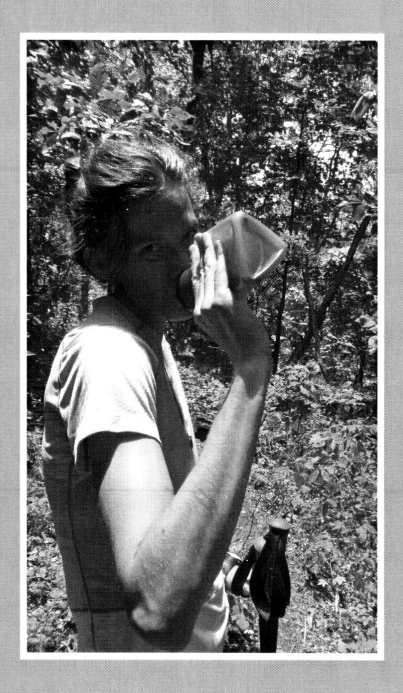

DAY 23

46.9 MILES

Today was huge for Jen. It wasn't important because she hiked almost 47 miles; it was important because she got to shower for the first time in 6 days.

The thought of a shower must be great motivation for Jen because each of the past days when she thinks she's getting a shower (into Delaware Water Gap and today into Pine Grove), she hikes REALLY fast.

I met her at Hawk Mountain Road a little before 8 AM. Rambler knew about a side trail near the Windsor Furnace Shelter so we were able to hike in ⅓ of a mile with water and a coffee and Egg McMuffins from McDonald's. Water sources are pretty scarce throughout most of Pennsylvania so it's been great having either Rambler or Dutch hike some of the longer stretches with Jen and carry an extra bottle or two.

Dutch hiked down to Port Clinton with Jen while I picked up a few packages from the post office. (Thanks for the cookies, Miles and Sally! And thanks to Sarah Merrell and Diamond Brand for the Clif Bars and Honey Stingers!) He hiked with her out of Port Clinton for a few miles, too, before backtracking.

Jim and Dutch went to the Cabela's near Hamburg to get Dutch some new shoes. (He didn't think he'd be doing any more hiking so he threw his old ones away after he reached Katahdin several weeks ago.) I went to McDonald's to use the internet and buy an Angus Deluxe burger for Jen.

Three of Jen's six or seven meals today happened to be from McDonald's. She said this afternoon that she could be the

McDonald's equivalent of Jared from Subway. "I ate McDonald's three times a day and actually LOST weight, and all I had to do was hike 45 miles a day!"

We met Jen at PA 183 and she cruised on through to PA 501 then on to PA 645. From there, we headed down into Pine Grove and got a couple of cheap hotels for the night. Jen took about a 30-minute shower, got to shave her legs, and then went to bed early so she could get almost 7 hours of sleep. The rocks haven't been too bad and the weather's been pretty good so far in Pennsylvania. Thanks for continuing to send all the positive e-mails, posts, thoughts, and prayers our way.

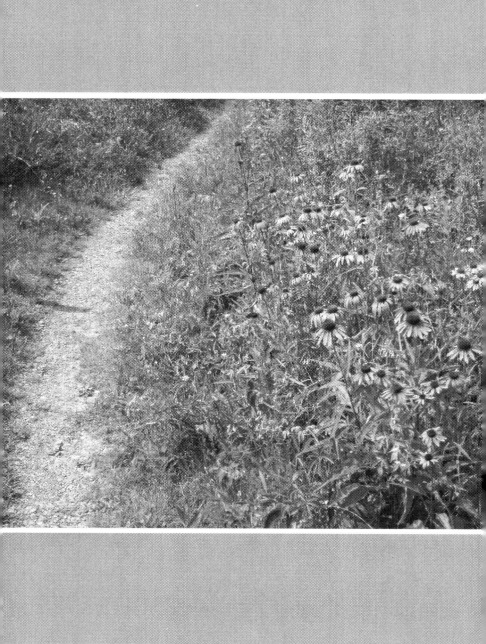

DAY 24
53.9 MILES

This was Jen's biggest mileage day since Day 1. Hiking this much is impressive enough in itself but doing it in a day-long rain through the rocks of Pennsylvania is even more impressive. She reached Swatara Gap around 8 AM and PA 443 about 25 minutes later. Jim hiked in a few miles with her pack so she wouldn't have to carry it quite so far on the 16-mile stretch, then Dutch hiked in from PA 325 to keep her company for the last mile or so. They got in around 12:45, so early that I was still napping. Rambler hiked in again with her pack for a few minutes before turning around, and Jen made it to PA 225 by about 4 PM.

Dutch and I went into Duncannon to shop for groceries, pick up some pizza, and check the internet, then we headed out to the Clarks Ferry Bridge and met up with Jen around 6:30. She and I road-walked into Duncannon together while Dutch drove my car around to meet up with Jim on the other side. From there, he and Jen hiked strong the last 8.5 miles to PA 850 and got in about 9:45.

Jen was really happy with her big day, but she can't get too complacent since it would be good for her to log another 50+ miler tomorrow over the relatively flat terrain of south central Pennsylvania around Carlisle, Boiling Springs, and Pine Grove Furnace State Park. Wow. I can't believe I'm married to this woman.

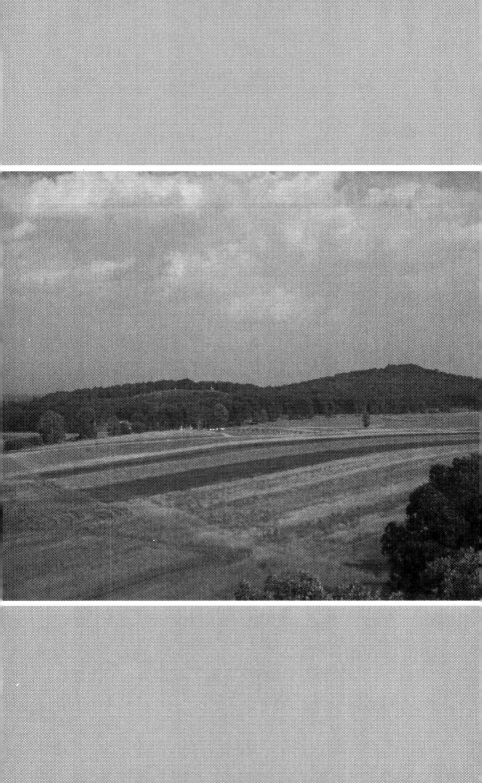

DAY 25
51.9 MILES

START TIME: 5:05 AM ✦ END TIME: 9:00 PM

Jen managed to put in another monster day. Rambler, Dutch, and I met her at Scott Farm around 7 AM. Rambler hiked with Jen for a short stretch before turning back around. He and Dutch met her at Trindle Road and he walked another 4 miles with her while I went into Carlisle to a pharmacy that sells a particular type of foam pre-wrap that Jen really likes for her feet and shins.

From there, Dutch and I drove to Boiling Springs, home of the Appalachian Trail Conservancy Mid-Atlantic Regional Office, and met up with Steve, who drove all the way down from Mahopac, New York, to hike a few more days with us. I walked the half-mile or so with Jen through Boiling Springs and Dutch hiked the next 10.6-mile stretch to Hunters Run Road.

Jim went into Carlisle and Steve and I drove past Mount Holly Springs to the home of Ryan and Jen Henry, two of Dave Horton's running buddies. Jen was out of town so Ryan was taking care of their two kids, but he invited us over for a visit so we could shower, do laundry, and eat a sandwich before heading back out to the trail.

Steve hiked the next 8.6-mile stretch with Jen to Pine Grove Furnace State Park. Jen's feet were hurting (I have no idea why . . .) so she soaked them in the creek near the parking lot while she ate Arby's chicken fingers and curly fries. Steve hiked a little farther with her before turning back, and Jen hiked alone the last 6 miles or so to Shippensburg Road. She arrived there around 7:15 PM. She and Dutch did the final stretch of 7.6 miles to Sandy Sod Junction in the Michaux State Forest. Rambler, Steve, and I drove to a little grocery store near Caledonia State Park where we got food for dinner. Jim picked up some Rocky Road ice cream so we could have a modified half gallon challenge.

If you're unfamiliar with the Appalachian Trail, the tradition is that when you cross the halfway point, which Jen did yesterday afternoon, you eat a half gallon of ice cream in an hour or so at the Pine Grove Furnace General Store. We didn't want Jen to get sick so we all pitched in and helped her finish it. It was another great day on the trail, and we definitely had reason to celebrate. Let's hope tomorrow goes just as well.

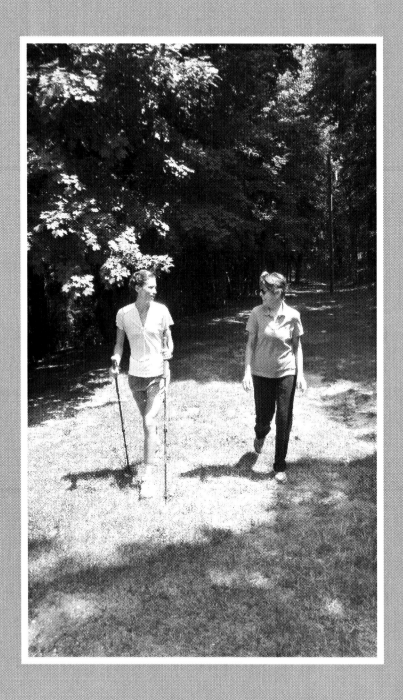

DAY 26
52.9 MILES

This was the third monster day in a row for Little Jen. She had been hoping to take advantage of these relatively flat miles in the Mid-Atlantic States and so far she's done exactly that. She left Sandy Sod Junction around 5 AM. I met her at US 30 near Caledonia State Park a little after 6 with a big cup of coffee and a breakfast burrito. The coffee and some sort of breakfast protein have become a routine the past week. Those and the protein shakes seem to help her get going in the early morning hours.

Rambler and Dutch met me at US 30 and Rambler hiked the next 4.7 miles with Jen. Steve got a cheap hotel just west of the state park and met up with us at PA 233 where he covered the next 10.6 miles with her. We met them a couple of times on some back roads before they came out on PA 16. Jen hiked the next 2.8 with Dutch and reached Pen-Mar Park on the Pennsylvania-Maryland border around noon.

Jen's Aunt Vee and Uncle Dudley had driven over from Leesburg, Virginia, for a special visit. Aunt Vee went running down the trail to give Jen a big hug when she saw her. They brought lots of treats for Jen and the Pit Crew: guacamole, tortilla chips, smoothies, blueberries, strawberries, bananas, and brownies. Jen was really encouraged by the visit. We had a perfect lunch looking out over the valley toward Hagerstown.

From Pen-Mar Park, Jen and Jim hiked 5.7 miles to Raven Rock Hollow, and Jen and Dutch hiked to MD 17. Steve drove home to New York from there after spending the better part of a week with us.

At MD 17, Jim joined her again for an 8.6-mile stretch to the I-70 footbridge, where I got to hike the last ³⁄₁₀ of a mile with her. She reached the Dahlgren Backpack Campground around 7 PM. I think Dahlgren is the only campground on the trail that has a free HOT shower. Jen had been looking forward to it for days.

After the shower, she and Dutch night-hiked the final 7.4-mile stretch to Gathland State Park.

For the record, Jen has hiked 158.7 miles in the past three days. That's over two marathons a day . . . for three days straight . . . on 6 hours of sleep a night. As Vizzini would say in *The Princess Bride*, "Inconceivable!" (Did I just quote *The Princess Bride*? You're darn right I did.)

super powers: At one of the road crossings today, Jen was explaining to the guys that she hikes best when she's had at least 7 hours of sleep or when she has a shower to look forward to at the end of the day (like today). She decided she'd start referring to these secret weapons as "7-hour power" and "shower power."

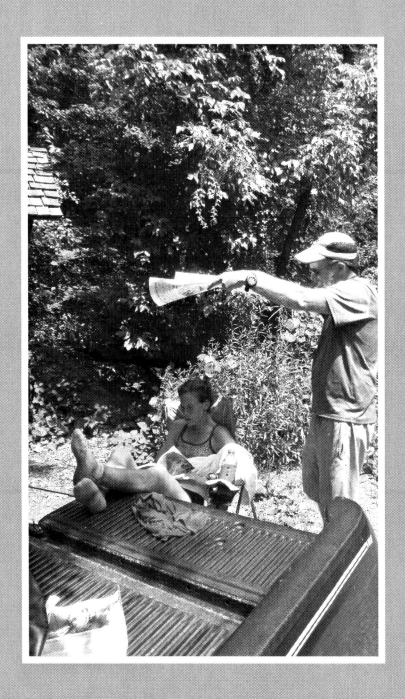

DAY 27
50.2 MILES

START TIME: 5:00 AM ✦ END TIME: 9:45 PM

It was very hot today. Well into the 90s. Horton and I both said we'd never seen Jen sweat so much. Still, she put in another 50-mile day. Her 4th in a row.

Jim and Dutch continued to hike big stretches with Jen. I got to hike the C&O Canal Towpath with her about 3 miles into Harper's Ferry. Dutch hiked the Roller Coaster with her. For those who don't know, it's a 13.5-mile stretch of continuous ups and downs. It's supposed to be really tough. They did it in the mid-afternoon heat but still cranked it out at a fast pace (probably 3.3 mph or so). It was the first time I'd seen Dutch look tired. He came in and grabbed a big chunk of ice out of the cooler and started putting it on her shoulders and neck. Jen just wore shorts and her sports bra for several stretches.

The end of the day was really tricky because they'd either have to hike in with gear (which would have slowed them down a lot) or the Pit Crew had to find a way to get in to them without any easily accessible road crossings. We managed to find one access point and it worked out perfectly. We reached the trail right as Jen and Dutch were hiking up, Jen ate her mac and cheese, and then hit the sack.

Jim will leave tomorrow, which is a real bummer because he's been an amazing asset. He knew the Pennsylvania trails incredibly well (I called him Warren Lite), he's a very strong hiker, and he's been willing to help out in any way he can. Dutch is planning on leaving on Friday to go sightseeing in

Washington, DC. Jen keeps asking him to stay. I keep saying, "I'm not going to try to influence you, Dutch. You need to do what you want." Really, though, I'm just playing the good cop to Jen's bad cop. We're hoping he'll forget about seeing the rest of the East Coast and just stay with us.

funny story: Before we got on the C&O Canal Towpath, we were talking about how easy that stretch should be because it has no elevation gain. Jen said, "I love the C&O Towpath. It's just like me: flat and fast." For those of you who don't know, Jen doesn't have the biggest boobs in the world.

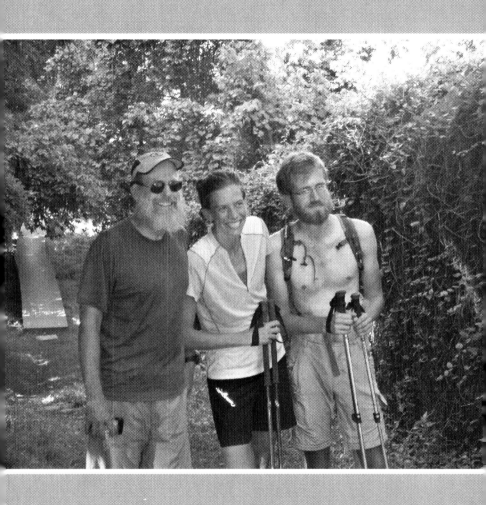

DAY 28

52.1 MILES

STAR TIME: 5:05 AM ✦ END TIME: 9:45 PM

This was Jen's fifth 50+ mile day in a row. She reached her first road (VA 55) about 7 AM and hiked the next 8.2-mile stretch with Rambler before he headed home to Amber, Pennsylvania.

We're bummed Rambler had to leave. He was a fantastic Pit Crew member. He was really efficient during Jen's road stops and I'm pretty sure he only took one shower while he was with us, so he fit in perfectly. Also, he's an awesome hiker.

At the end of the next 5.6-mile stretch, Jen and Dutch reached Skyline Drive in Shenandoah National Park. Jen's been looking forward to SNP because it's relatively easy hiking and there are road crossings about every three miles so she can just camel up at the car and not carry any food and water. Also, she digs animals, and there are a lot of those here. She calls it the "Shenandoah Petting Zoo." It's not quite a petting zoo, but it's close. Jen saw a couple of bears today, and when I pulled into the Skyland Lodge parking lot there were "Don't Feed the Animals" signs everywhere. There were also deer lounging around within yards of the hotel guests.

Jen put up big miles again because the weather wasn't as hot as yesterday. Also, she was tapping into her "shower power." She saw in the data book that if she could put in 52 miles, then we could stay at the Skyland Lodge and she could get clean again. When she found out our room had a tub and that she could take her first bath in over a month, she was even happier.

By nightfall, she was definitely feeling the string of 50-mile days. She felt better after bathing and she was happy to sleep in a real bed, but again, she's going to have to turn around and do it all over again tomorrow so she can't get complacent.

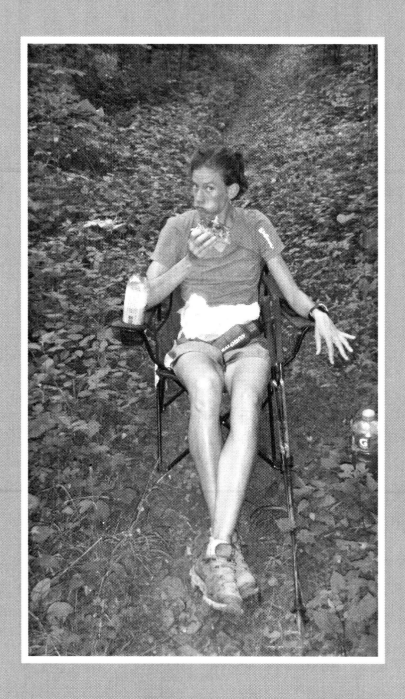

DAY 29

46.8 MILES

START TIME: 6:15 AM ✦ END TIME: 9:30 PM

Today, Jen did something no one else on an AT speed record attempt has EVER done before. Not Warren. Not Horton. Not Pete Palmer. Not Andrew Thompson. Not Karl. All of those guys are AMAZING hikers, but none of them has ever . . . ever . . . taken a pregnancy test.

That's right. Jen woke up at 4:45 this morning and for the 3rd day in a row, she felt queasy. Like "morning sickness" queasy. We went out to the trail a little after 5, but she felt so sick that she decided to go back to the lodge and sleep an extra hour.

I was a little worried. The queasiness could have been from the 5 consecutive 50+ mile days or it could have been from the intense heat two days ago. Or it could have been something we ate. Or from the hotel room itself. Because I felt a little queasy, too. Or it could have been that she was pregnant.

So Horton picked up a kit on the way to the trail and she took it at the second road crossing. You'll be happy to know (all of you except our parents) that the stick said "not pregnant." Jen said that's probably the last time she'll be happy to find that out. At least until we're, like, 50 or something.

Because of the late start and especially because of the queasiness, I wasn't sure if she would get many miles in today. But she started feeling better as the day progressed. One thing that helped a TON was that she had a record "bear" day.

During her first thru-hike in 2005, Jen didn't see any bears. During her 2008 record attempt, she saw thirty of them. And today alone, she saw 14! Horton couldn't believe it. Several times she saw a momma bear with two cubs. Once she saw a daddy bear by himself and another time she saw a couple of older siblings with no momma. It really encouraged her to see all wildlife, and I guess it reinforces the fact that there are TONS of animals in Shenandoah National Park, which kind of makes sense because probably no other national park is as surrounded by humans as SNP, so the animals have nowhere else to go.

food: Horton got a couple of stuffed crust pizzas from Pizza Hut. I was skeptical (just like I was skeptical when he brought the McGriddles from McDonald's. A sandwich made of pancakes? Please . . .), but it was actually very good. We also enjoyed blackberry milkshakes and my friend Miles's famous cookies (he sent 5 or 6 dozen) in addition to the usual fare. Jen continues to get as many liquid calories as possible from smoothies, protein shakes, fruit juices, ice cream, chocolate milk, you name it. She's at the point where she gags whenever she starts eating solid foods at the road crossings, so she's much happier when she doesn't have to chew.

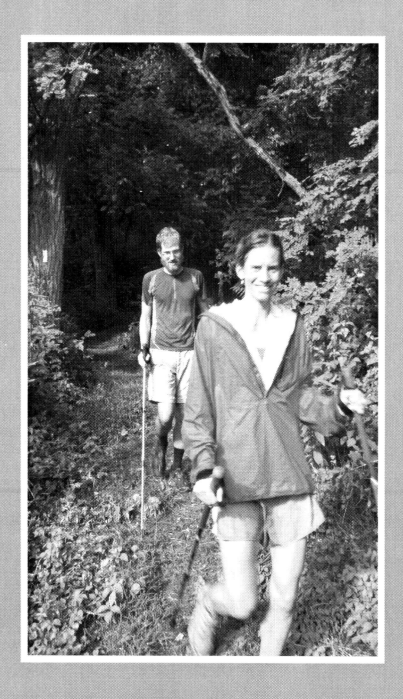

DAY 30
52.9 MILES

START TIME: 5:05 AM ✦ END TIME: 9:40 PM

I was worried that Jen would feel nauseous again this morning, but you can see from her miles that she felt just fine. No pregnancy test needed today!

She didn't have another record "bear" day—she "only" saw 2—but the Pit Crew set our own sort of personal record. By my calculations, we managed to meet Jen at 14 different road crossings, 10 of them before noon. I mentioned in an earlier blog that the AT crosses Skyline Drive every 3 or 4 miles. Well, this morning it crossed it about every 2. So Jen didn't have to carry anything. She just took pit-stops every hour or so. Most were short, but a few were longer.

In the mid-morning, Horton donned the mantle of Pit Crew Chief for a few hours so I could go into Waynesboro to shower, pick up a package, run by the bank, shop for groceries, and get lunch from Shukri's BBQ.

When I got back on the Blue Ridge Parkway at Rockfish Gap, where Shenandoah National Park ends, I met Horton at the side trail to the Humpback Rocks Visitor Center and we hiked in to meet Jen and Dutch. After they ate some BBQ, they hiked another 8 miles to the Dripping Rock Parking Area.

Horton drove home to Lynchburg from there, and Dutch took about a 5-mile break before hiking the final 10.7-mile stretch with Jen from Reeds Gap to VA 56. They left about 6:40 so I wasn't expecting to see them until after 10, but they cruised in at 9:37.

Dutch is leaving tomorrow. The past few days, Jen has worn his Ace ankle bandage, in part because of her shin splints but mostly because she thinks Dutch's speed hiking powers will rub off on her that way. She says he's a faster hiker than me. I find that hard to believe.

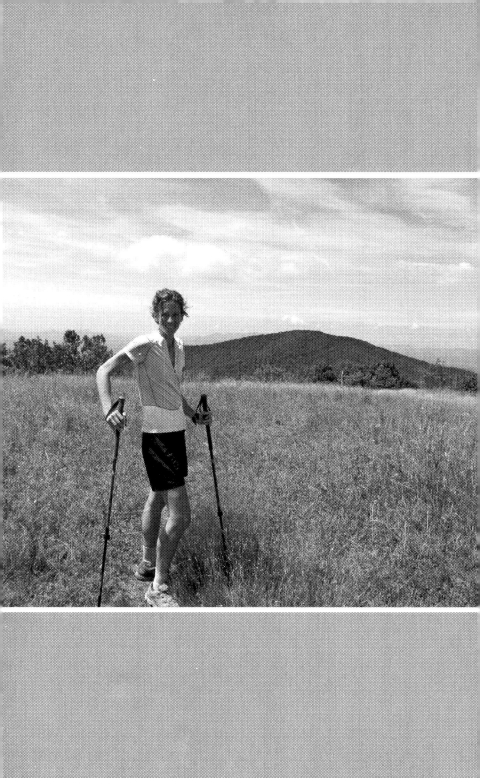

DAY 31

49.7 MILES

START TIME: 5:00 AM ✦ END TIME: 9:25 PM

Today turned out to be another day of transitions. We didn't have nearly the number of people coming and going as we did in Palmerton, but these transitions were just as significant.

Dutch camped out with us last night by the Tye River. He and Jen were off at the crack of dawn to climb the Priest, which is probably the biggest climb Jen's had since Moosilauke in New Hampshire.

They made good time over it and reached Cash Hollow Road around 7 o'clock. Horton brought breakfast burritos and McMuffins from McDonald's, and yogurt and donut holes from his favorite gas station/convenience store Sheetz.

That was the last stretch Dutch hiked with Jen before heading to DC for a week of sightseeing. We tried to tell him there's nothing to see there, but he didn't buy it. So Horton drove him to Charlottesville where he boarded a train.

We were incredibly fortunate to have Dutch with us for a week and a half, and we hope to see him again sometime. Maybe he'll join us if we go hiking in Europe next summer.

When Dutch left, David Horton left, too. He finished a mountain bike race that ran the length of the Rockies about a week ago so he was zonked and missing his wife and grandkids. We agreed that it was best for him to be in Lynchburg with them.

But he connected us with another ultra runner from Lynchburg named Rebecca Trittapoe. Jen knows Rebecca from the race circuit and felt good about having her with us. She met us at Salt Log Gap around 10:30 this morning and so far she's been an awesome addition. She and Jen seem to have great conversations while they hike. Even though Rebecca's recovering from a knee injury, she's very capable of keeping up with Jen for big stretches of trail.

Last night, I tried to trick Jen into another 50-mile day. Let me explain . . . On her 2008 hike, I bungled a road crossing one morning in Maine and she ended up having to put in 38 miles with no re-supply. When I finally met her at dusk, I said jokingly that I'd missed her on purpose because I wanted her to do an extra 10 miles. Hysterical, right?

From then on, anytime I missed her by accident, we joked that I was trying to trick her into hiking more miles.

So the goal at the beginning of the day was to make VA 501/130 near the James River Foot Bridge. When Jen reached Punchbowl Mountain Crossing about 11 miles out, she told me she wanted to camp 1.5 miles past the road at a campsite that was listed in the databook. I remembered camping near the James River in 2008, but I didn't remember whether there was a shelter at the site or not.

Because of my knee injury I haven't really "hiked in" yet this year, but this was a flat stretch and I had plenty of time to take it slow. Well, I reached the campsite after only 30 minutes and I didn't feel like I'd been hiking 3 mph. Also, there's no camping for a mile along the river and the site was really close to the river so I assumed it was an illegal one.

I pressed on hoping to come across the real campsite but about 15 minutes later I ended up walking into Matts Creek Shelter, 2.3 miles from the road. I was worried that Jen might be wiped out and not want to take another step past the campsite, but she and Rebecca missed it, too. It all worked out because I set up the tent at the shelter and brought food back so Jen could eat on the trail. And the first thing she said when she saw me was, "Were you trying to trick me into a 50 mile day?" Yes. Yes I was.

animal sightings: Jen saw two more bears today. I haven't kept count but if she hasn't seen 30 yet (the number she saw on her 2008 hike), she's definitely getting close.

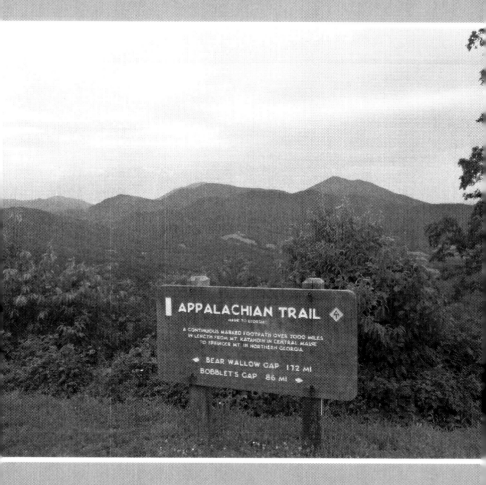

DAY 32
52.6 MILES

START TIME: 5:05 AM   ✦   END TIME: 10:15 PM

For the 7th time in 9 days, Jen hiked over 50 miles. She left Matts Creek Shelter before dawn and Rebecca and I slept another 45 minutes or so before packing up and hiking the 2 miles back to VA 501. I drove into Big Island to pick up breakfast sandwiches and coffee while Rebecca drove around to meet Jen at Petites Gap.

For most of the day, we were able to see her every few miles as she crisscrossed the Blue Ridge Parkway. She did have one or two longer stretches, and Rebecca would hike in on those. But for the first half of the day, we were seeing her about every hour.

One thing that made the day more fun for Jen, Rebecca, and me was that we ran into some guys from Lynchburg—Jeremy Ramsey, Frank Gonzalez, and Kevin (I didn't catch Kevin's last name)—who were doing a 30-mile training run along the AT. They ran into Jen a couple of times, chatted with her, and sat with us at some of road crossings. It was pretty cool hearing these elite trail runners—guys who were out for a 30 mile *training* run—talking about what a freak of nature Jen was.

A little later in the day, I was turning around in the middle of a gravel road when a mountain biker in a funny-looking unitard came careening down the hill. I started to apologize for blocking him then I realized it was Horton. He'd ridden 78 miles round-trip from Lynchburg to say "hi" and hang out for a few minutes. The guy just finished mountain biking 120 miles a day for almost a month on the Western Continental

Divide and he's back on his bike already. What a wingnut. (Kidding, Horton. Sort of . . .)

Later in the day, another Lynchburg trail runner named Gratton Garboe brought us a spaghetti dinner and turned out to be a big help with some logistical issues.

here's what happened: There was a little-used forest road that was gated near the Blue Ridge Parkway. I drove around to access it because it fell in the middle of a 13-mile section and because Horton provoked me by saying Kadrah couldn't find it when she was crewing Adam. So, of course, I accepted the challenge and went looking for it. And I found it.

But the drive up was gnarly and it took a long time, and I didn't want to make a second trip. Fortunately, I had cell phone service and Gratton, who'd already found the girls, had his phone on. I got in touch with him and Rebecca and told them I was staying put and that they should send Jen on.

Jen and Rebecca got to eat some of the spaghetti that Gratton had brought, but I didn't (since, you know, I was proving my masculinity and all by finding a road) so he was nice enough to run down from the Parkway to deliver dinner and keep me company for a while.

Jen came through around 8:05. She was talking about how tough the last stretch was, so we decided that she should stop at Fullhardt Knob Shelter. Rebecca was already hiking in from Mountain Pass Road to meet her and either camp at the shelter or hike the last 3 miles to VA 652.

Right as Jen was leaving, I said I was getting a hotel room in Daleville and that she could shower there when she came out in the morning. Well, about ten minutes after Gratton headed back to his car and I headed down the mountain, Jen called and said in this exaggerated sad, whiny, self-aware voice that she sometimes uses after hiking 50 miles a day, "*I want to* stay in the hotel with *you* . . . and *I* want to sleep in a bed and *I* want to take a shower . . . This [carrying an overnight pack] is an inefficient use of my *energy.* . . . I'm only three miles from the road . . ." It was really pathetic . . . but cute, too.

Down the mountain, there was another defunct road that we thought might lead up to the trail, but we hadn't tried to use it because we weren't sure. I'd already started hiking up it to surprise Jen. So when she called, I was able to find her, take her pack, and let her keep going down the mountain. Then about five minutes after Jen and I ran into each other, we ran into Rebecca.

On hikes like this, every now and then, you have these significant moments where you experience the essence of endurance hiking. Seeing Jen and Warren cross the Kennebec was one of those moments. Watching Jen dance and scream the Mumford & Sons line, "I'll find STRENGTH IN PAIN," when she finished the Whites was another. And having Rebecca and me converge to meet her when she really needed it was a third.

Endurance hikes aren't for everyone. They're a different sort of experience. But after being out here for over a month, I'm convinced that you can draw just as much meaning from them and from the relationships you create during them as from a traditional thru-hike. You just have to know where to look.

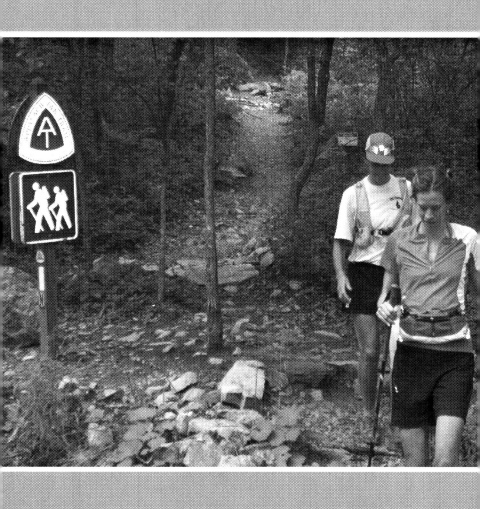

DAY 33
46.9 MILES

START TIME: 5:35 AM ✦ END TIME: 10:10 PM

Last night, I told Jen we could get a hotel room only if she promised to get at least 6 hours of sleep. She agreed so we "slept in" until 5:15. We were at VA 652 by 5:35 and she hiked the two miles down to US 220 by 6:20.

Jen's college professor, advisor, and friend, Doug Clapp, was staying at Smith Mountain Lake for the weekend with his wife, Sarah, and some grad school friends, and he wanted to come out and hike a few miles with Jen. At first the plan was for them to hike the flat 2-mile stretch between 652 and 220, but Doug would have had to wake up even earlier to do that so he hiked up to Tinker Ridge with Jen instead. It's a much tougher climb but they did it early enough in the day that the heat wasn't a factor, which was really important because it's a very long, very dry stretch.

Around 7:30, Rebecca hiked up from a side trail about 10 miles in so Jen wouldn't have to get off the ridge for water or carry 20 miles worth of it.

Rebecca hiked with Jen three or four more times throughout the day, and then carried most of her stuff in at dusk so they could have a "girls' night"—that's what Jen called it—between VA 621 and VA 630.

Rebecca has been a great Pit Crew member. She doesn't smell bad, and she showered at least once while she was with us, so that's a strike against her. But she knows the trails in this part of Virginia, she's tough and in shape, she entertained Jen with stories of her trail running adventures, and she did everything she could to make Jen comfortable. She's heading back to Lynchburg tomorrow morning. We're grateful she was willing to help out these past three days.

funny story: This morning Jen said she feels like she's becoming a toddler again. She sips Juicy Juice and chocolate milk from lidded plastic bottles. She's picky about what she eats. She gets cranky when she's tired (but to be honest, she's always done that). She prefers pureed or mushy food instead of solid food. And she uses Wet Wipes all the time.

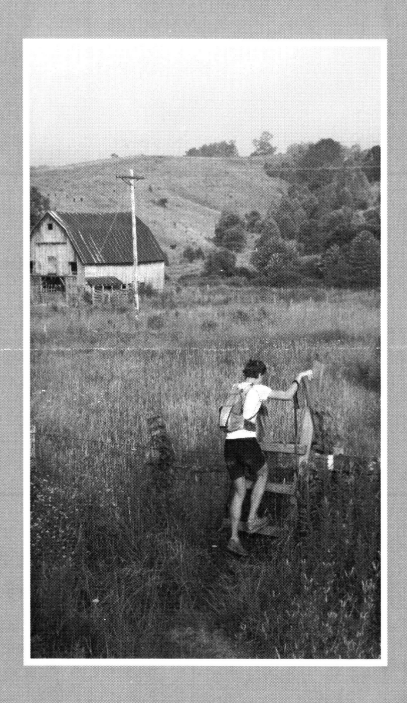

DAY 34
47.3 MILES

START TIME: 5:15 AM ✦ END TIME: 8:55 PM

Today was a great day. Jen was able to reach Pearisburg over some really difficult terrain.

She woke up at the usual time and made it down to VA 630 by 7:35. I camped at the trailhead, which was a good thing because Jen got there at least 30 minutes earlier than I'd expected. I'd just finished making her a ham and cheese sandwich when she rolled in.

Rebecca hiked back to her car at VA 621 when Jen woke up, then drove around to give me the pack, tent, and the rest of the gear at VA 42. After that, she headed home to Lynchburg. (BIG shout out to Rebecca for her help these last three days. Thanks, Rebecca!)

At the next road crossing, Rocky Gap, which was 5.4 miles down the trail, an ATC "Trails to Every Classroom" group was doing some GPS work, which was neat because Jen had worked with the same program in North Carolina this past spring.

From there, she had a 2.1-mile stretch down to Johns Creek Valley, then a 5.9-mile stretch to Mountain Lake Road. And *that*, my friends, is where we met up with the legendary Matt Kirk, his wife, Lily, and their dog, Uwharrie.

Matt is a stud. I don't know any other word to describe him. In recent years, he has set endurance records on the Benton MacKaye Trail, the Mountains-to-Sea Trail, and the South Beyond 6,000 (SB6K) summits. He's hiked the AT twice and has done some other crazy stuff like run 100 miles through Shenandoah National Park in 24 hours.

Lily is no slouch, either. She thru-hiked the AT in 2007. And their dog, Uwharrie, (named for the national forest in North Carolina where Matt found her)—well, Uwharrie has four legs so she was born to run.

As soon as Jen re-fueled at Mountain Lake Road, she, Matt, and Uwharrie headed out. They covered the first 7.1 miles in less than 2.5 hours.

Then they *really* started moving. The three of them completed the rocky, dry, 17.6-mile stretch from Stony Creek Valley to Clendenin Road near Pearisburg in five hours and fifteen minutes.

I couldn't believe it. I mean Jen has covered some stretches really fast on this hike, but nothing like that. When I saw them, I said, "Wow! That was *crazy* fast!" Jen grinned, raised her poles over her head for emphasis, and yelled, "I know, right?! *Matt-freakin'-Kirk's* here!"

From there, Lily and I drove the cars across the bridge and walked back toward them. Then we all had a leisurely stroll over the Senator Shumate Bridge.

The human hikers scarfed down the tacos and enchiladas we'd gotten them, and the canine hiker scarfed down dog food. After that, we drove to the Holiday Motor Lodge where Jen showered, doctored her feet, and climbed into bed early.

Over the past two days, Jen has averaged 47.1 miles. I think most folks who are familiar with this particular stretch of the AT would agree that hiking from Daleville to Pearisburg in two days is as hard or harder than all those 50-mile days she put in through Pennsylvania, Maryland, and the Shenandoahs.

Positive thoughts and prayers: Jen and I were talking last night about how this is a tough spot on the trail, not so much because of the terrain—although the terrain is certainly not easy—but because we've been out for a long time (well over a month), but we're still not in the home stretch. And that means we're feeling pretty fatigued mentally and physically. We appreciate the positive thoughts and prayers you have sent our way to help us deal with that. Thanks!

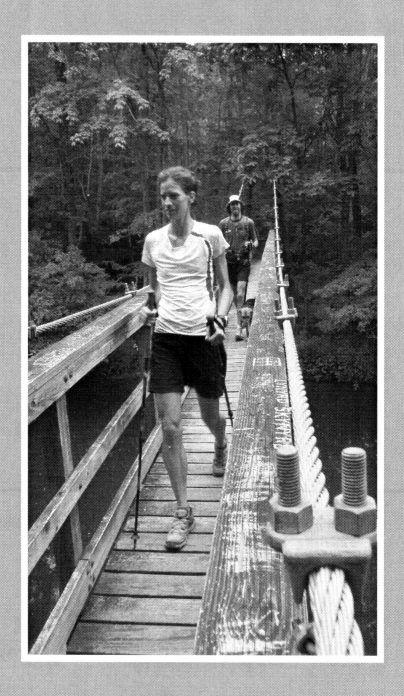

DAY 35
50.3 MILES

START TIME: 5:15 AM ✦ END TIME: 9:25 PM

I'm really proud of Jen for completing another 50-mile day. In 2008, she did 65 miles on her last full day, but didn't have another one above 47. This time, I think she's completed eight.

After she set off from the Senator Shumate Bridge at 5:15, I went back to the hotel for another hour of sleep. At around 7 o'clock, Matt and Lily ran to Hardee's for some breakfast sandwiches while I cleaned out Jen's water bottles.

I don't think I've mentioned this, but Jen's water bottles get nasty. After a few hours in the heat, the juice ferments and has a real kick to it.

We were supposed to meet Jen 10.9 miles in at Sugar Run Gap but I went to Big Horse Gap instead, which was 1.6 miles south. It worked out fine, though. Jen kept hiking like she was supposed to. Matt had run in to meet her and they ran into each other somewhere in the middle.

They took a short break at Big Horse Gap, enough time for Jen to wolf down a bacon, egg, and cheese biscuit and chug some chocolate milk, then they headed out for the next 12.3-mile stretch. I should mention that Uwharrie did not accompany them on this first stretch. She was noticeably depressed hanging out with Lily and me, but she did get to run quite a few miles later in the day.

Jen and Matt arrived at VA 606 at 1:20 and took another 20-minute break before heading toward Lickskillet Hollow (probably my favorite road crossing name so far). Jen was feeling really sleepy when she got there. She thought maybe it was because she'd eaten a second bacon, egg, and cheese biscuit at the last road crossing, and that's a little heavier than what she normally eats for lunch.

At any rate, she was wide awake by the time she reached the next road crossing, VA 611, because the carcass of a deer was rotting about ten feet from the road and the trail and was emitting the most heinous stench imaginable. It was so bad that Lily drove her car 50 yards past the road crossing to escape it. So bad that Jen and Matt said they could smell it hundreds of yards away.

When they left for the second to last stretch of the day—8.2 miles to VA 612 near I-77—Lily and I headed into Bland (that's right, Bland), Virginia, to go grocery shopping. I was disappointed, but not surprised, to find that the only grocery store in town, the one I'd visited during Jen's 2008 hike, had closed down.

And instead of driving 20 miles to the nearest grocery store in Wytheville, we decided to try Dollar General instead.

I don't know how many of you have been to Dollar General recently, but it was actually the perfect place for me to resupply because it has just about everything except fresh produce, and Jen and I practically took an oath to eat nothing but processed foods for the duration of the trip. I can picture Jen's mom, and her Aunt Vee, and cousin Tori rolling their eyes right now. But the sad truth is, fruits and vegetables take too much time and energy to chew. They have a lot of sugar but not enough calories, so they're kind of a waste of time on a hike like this. I've been trying to eat a banana or apple or *something* healthy every day. But the only fruit that Jen's gotten is from fruit smoothies and the only vegetables she's gotten are in potato chips.

When Lily and I arrived at VA 612, we couldn't believe what we found. Or rather smelled: *another* dead animal. We thought the first one had been a coincidence, but after the second one, we decided someone around here didn't like thru-hikers.

Jen, Matt, and Uwharrie arrived at VA 612 around 7:30, and I got to do a .8-mile road walk over I-77 with Jen. At US 52, Matt and Uwharrie rejoined her and the three of them cranked out the last 7.7 miles to VA 615 in about two hours and fifteen minutes. We found a couple of great campsites by the river. Jen was able to eat her Mountain House, take her usual Wet Wipe bath, and hit the sack by 10:15 or so.

We want to give a BIG shout out to uber-hiker Matt Kirk— and another BIG shout out to his wife Lily—for their willingness to join us for a couple of days on the tail end of their vacation to West Virginia. Matt helped Jen out a lot, especially that first day into Pearisburg. And I really enjoyed hanging out with Lily, even if we were often surrounded by the rotting flesh of dead animals.

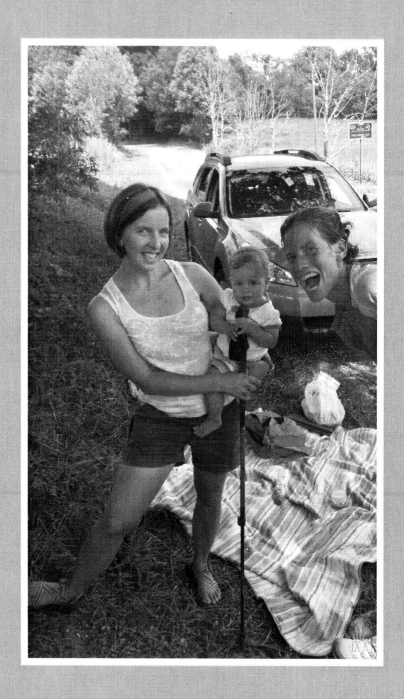

DAY 36

49.2 MILES

START TIME: 5:05 AM ✦ END TIME: 9:35 PM

Jen had another great day, partly because she put in nearly 50 miles, but mostly because she got to see our little niece, Hazel, for the first time in about 6 weeks. That's because Jen's brother, James, and his wife, Lindsay, drove up with Hazel and met us at VA 42 around 1 o'clock.

But Jen got about 8 hours of hiking in before they arrived so I should probably start there. She woke up at 4:45 like she always does. One thing I haven't mentioned is that she's waking up at the same time, but she's hiking before sunrise since we're further south and the summer equinox was about a month ago. When she began in Maine, the sky was just starting to lighten when she got on the trail, but now she hikes with a headlamp for a solid hour before dawn.

She made it to Garden Mountain by 7:55 or so. That's on the south ridge of Burke's Garden, which is this enigmatic little valley in southwest Virginia. The locals call it "God's Thumbprint" and if you've never seen it, it's worth a visit on a clear day. But this was not a clear day. There was thick fog and cloud-cover for most of the morning.

For breakfast, Jen had a sausage, egg, and cheese biscuit and a coffee from the Citgo in Bland (haute cuisine at its finest). While she was eating, I took a picture of her new shoes: lime green Synapses from Salomon. Then she took five or six dietary supplement pills that she's been taking since Katahdin.

I know what you're thinking. No, they're not performance

enhancing drugs. We don't dope, either. She's just a freak of nature. Plain and simple.

But recently, Jen's been gagging on the pills because they're kind of big. I, of course, have tried to say logical things like, "Maybe you should take two at a time instead of an entire handful." But the same determination that allows her to hike 45-50 miles a day also compels her to shove ridiculous amounts of pills in her mouth all at once.

Anyway, she ended up puking. I gave her a Wet Wipe and after she'd cleaned off her face and legs, she said in a cheerful, sing-songy voice, "It looked like a beautiful waterfall." Then, ever the pragmatist, she said, "Well, I guess it's good you took a picture of the shoes *before* I threw up on them."

Then about 30 seconds after she'd cleaned up and taken a swig of water, she was back on the trail. What a woman.

She made it to Walker Gap on the southwest corner of Burke's Garden by 9:55 and she reached VA 42 west of Ceres around 1:40. She flew through that 12.4-mile section in about three hours and forty minutes. That's because she knew our niece was going to be at the road crossing. When Jen saw us all standing there, she came running down the trail with her hands out yelling, "Hazel! Hazel!" She was on kind of a steep descent so I had to tell her to slow down.

For the next fifteen minutes, she alternated between holding Hazel, drinking chocolate milk, and eating a roast beef wrap. Then she and James headed out for a 2.4-mile stretch to VA 610 then a 9.4 mile-stretch to US 11.

Lindsay, Hazel, and I ran a few errands and went to our respective hotels before heading back to the trail around 5 o'clock. Warren and Teri Doyle drove up from Mountain City, Tennessee, to surprise Jen, so we sat around and visited with them until Jen and James arrived at 5:35 or so. Jen did a

2.7-mile stretch to the Settlers Museum in Atkins by herself and then James hiked the final 8.8 miles with her.

I went back into town with Lindsay to make some calls and send some e-mails, then I went to Taco Bell for our dinner. There were a lot of restaurant choices in Marion, but we ate Taco Bell the last time we were here so I thought Jen might appreciate the nostalgia of it. Besides Marion, I think we've only eaten at a Taco Bell one other time. She wolfed down three soft tacos and chugged some chocolate milk on the way back to the hotel, then she took a shower and hit the sack around 10:45.

You may notice that we're staying in more hotels the further south we get. The obvious reason for that is Jen digs the showers. It's clear after today, though, that she benefits from "Hazel power" as much as "shower power."

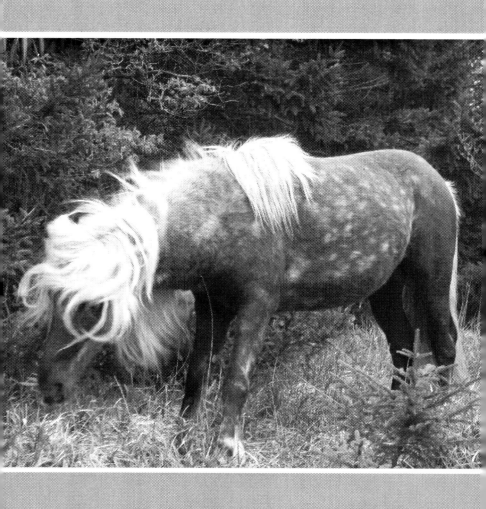

DAY 37
46.9 MILES

START TIME: 5:25 AM   ✦   END TIME: 8:45 PM

Jen crossed over one of her favorite stretches of the trail today: Grayson Highlands State Park in southwest Virginia. She got started a bit later than usual because we stayed at a hotel in Marion and because it took us a few extra minutes to find the trailhead in the dark. Once she got started, though, she made great time. She reached VA 670 (South Fork of the Holston River) by 7:45 and Dickey Gap a little before 10.

Rambler came down from Pennsylvania to rejoin the Pit Crew for a few days. He met me at Dickey Gap, hiked in a short ways to see Jen, then hiked the next 8.5 miles with her to VA 603 at Fox Creek. James, Lindsay, and Hazel also met us at Dickey Gap, and they brought breakfast burritos, sausage McMuffins, coffee, and chocolate milk for Jen's second breakfast of the morning.

James, Lindsay, and I drove to VA 603 and lounged around on a picnic blanket while Hazel kept trying to grab dirt and eat leaves. It's obvious she already loves the woods, and that she's going to be a hiker when she grows up.

When Jen and Rambler arrived, James took Rambler's place and hiked with Jen for the next 9.8 miles up to Massie Gap. While they were doing that, Lindsay, Hazel, and I grabbed lunch while Rambler went on to Massie Gap to "summit" Mt. Rogers (Virginia's highest point). "Summit" here is a relative term because there are probably a dozen unofficial summits of Mt. Rogers.

After eating and checking e-mail, Lindsay, Hazel, and I

drove to Grayson Highlands and climbed up from the Massie Gap parking lot to meet Jen and James. They arrived about 3:45 and took a short break before heading down to VA 600 and Elk Garden.

Aside from the sleet and rain in the Whites, and the scorching heat in Maryland, Jen's been very fortunate with weather so far, and today was no exception. About the time she and James rolled into Elk Garden (6:10 or so), we could hear and see a massive thunderstorm off in the distance toward Grayson Highlands.

Rambler hiked the last stretch of the day with Jen down to US 58, while James and Lindsay helped me shuttle Rambler's car around before they headed home.

Jen only saw three ponies today, and they are a big reason why she loves Grayson Highlands so much. But she didn't seem too disappointed about it. Holding our 9-month-old niece is probably the only thing that could make Jen happier than petting the Grayson Highland ponies.

two random thoughts: First, James did a *great* job hiking with Jen. In the roughly 30 hours he was with us, he covered 35 miles with her.

Second, Lily Kirk suggested I take the Highlander to get a car wash. I weighed the pros and cons, and eventually determined that I was going to take the Manny Ramirez approach. For those of you who don't follow baseball, Manny Ramirez was a quirky slugger for the Indians, Red Sox, and Dodgers who refused to clean his batting helmet. It was covered with dirt, tar, sweat, and no telling what else, but he insisted on keeping it filthy until the end of the season when the Red Sox won the World Series.

Maybe I'm taking the Manny Ramirez approach because I'm hoping Jen will reach her goal, too. Or maybe I want the car to fit in with the rest of the Pit Crew. Or maybe I'm just being lazy. Regardless, there will be about 7 weeks' worth of dirt, oil, mud, and no telling what else on the Highlander when we reach Springer. Then, and only then, will it get a bath.

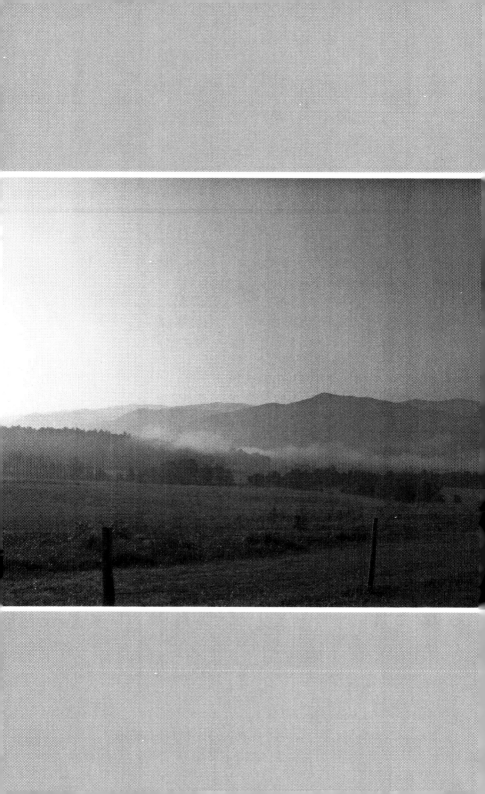

DAY 38

49.8 MILES

START TIME: 5:05 AM   ✦   END TIME: 9:50 PM

Jen had another near-50-mile day. She got a full 7 hours of
sleep last night before hitting the trail at the usual time. The
first road crossing was VA 728 but it was a little tougher to find
than we thought. That's because it was still dark when we got
out there and because the road didn't actually cross the trail; it
crossed OVER the trail. On an old train bridge. Rambler and I
knew we were close, and we knew the trail would eventually
meet the road we were walking in on, but we weren't sure how
far we'd have to walk. Once the railroad grade got low enough
for us to notice it, Rambler pointed out that the trail was probably up there. About 50 yards later, I spotted a white blaze on
a tree above us so we scrambled up the steep embankment and
hiked back toward the bridge. Jen made me promise not to
climb back down the embankment again. I didn't want to go
back down because of my knee and because of erosion, but I let
her feel like she'd won a big victory anyway.

Things were less eventful the rest of the day. Rambler hiked
a few miles in with Jen from VA 728 and then we both met her
at Straight Branch on US 58. From there she hiked 5.6 miles
into Damascus, one of the best towns on the trail.

I spent several hours in Damascus sending e-mails, making
phone calls, shopping for groceries, pizza, and flashlights,
doing laundry, talking with Warren—who had come over
from his home in Mountain City—and meeting up with Maureen, a friend of Jen's family from way back.

Rambler got a head start up the trail from Damascus and

carried Jen's water and snacks for the first part of the 15-mile stretch. Once he came back down, he, Maureen, and I drove around to Low Gap on US 421 near Shady Valley. Jen came through a little before 4 and ate some of the snacks Maureen brought from Lake Summit: watermelon, cantaloupe, and hard-boiled eggs from her chickens.

Once the three of us got to Tenn. 91, Maureen helped me clean out my trunk. I resisted but she said it was unhealthy to serve Jen food from such a filthy car. And I never meant for the Manny Ramirez approach to apply to the inside, just the outside. So I didn't put up a fight, especially when she yelled at me, "Let me be helpful!"

While we were cleaning out the trunk, a storm hit and dumped rain on us for 20 or 30 minutes. I was sure Jen would get soaked by it, but when she came strolling in, she didn't have a single drop on her.

From there, she had an 11.5-mile stretch to Vandeventer Shelter. Rambler, Maureen, and I drove around to Wilbur Dam Road, where Rambler hiked 4.7 miles in with Jen's tent, sleeping bag, pad, and dinner.

After he left, Maureen drove into Elizabethton to get a hotel room, I put up my tent, and within about 15 minutes, it was pouring again. At about 9:45, I got a text from Jen saying she'd made it safely. I called thinking we both might have reception, and we did so we were able to talk for a few minutes. It turned out she avoided the second storm, too, but she was sleeping close enough to the shelter that she could hear someone snoring loudly. We're not sure, but there's a decent chance it was Rambler.

retroactive animal sighting: I forgot to mention that Jen crossed paths with a big, mean rattlesnake several days ago. He was camped out in the trail at a forest road crossing. She kept her distance and whacked her sticks to try to get him to move.

She even started throwing stuff around him (not *at* him), but he didn't budge. He just coiled up and started rattling. After a few minutes, she decided to give him a wide berth and walked around him in the woods.

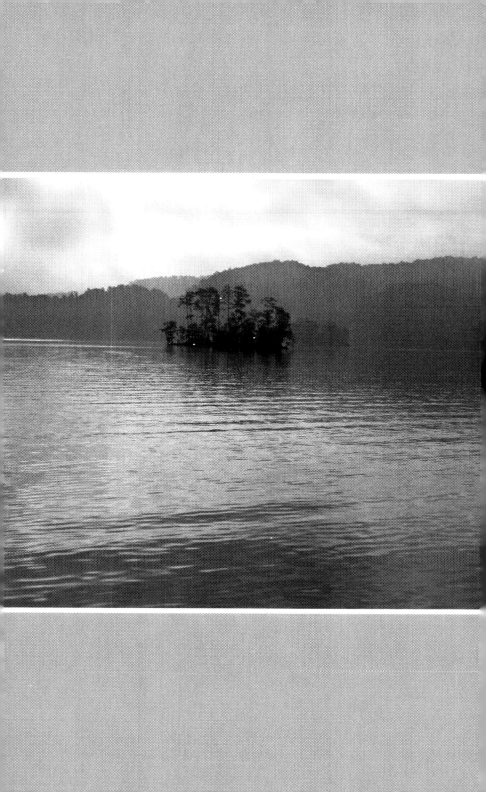

DAY 39

46.1 MILES

START TIME: 5:05 AM ✦ END TIME: 9:40 PM

Jen must be living right, because four really incredible things happened to her today.

The first was that she got stung by a bee. And she's allergic to bees. You're probably wondering, "How is that lucky?" Well, it's lucky because I happened to stick a couple of Benadryl in her little-used hip pack today, and I have NEVER put Benadryl in there before. So she was able to take the meds as soon as she got stung so it didn't affect her as much.

The second incredible thing was that the Pit Crew got caught in three substantial rain showers and one massive thunderstorm, but the little Hiker Princess came away unscathed. Not a single drop hit her.

Somewhere in one of the gospels, Jesus said, "the rain falls on the just and the unjust." So we've decided that Jen must be neither.

But the wet weather made for cooler temperatures, so Jen got to enjoy the benefits of the rain without any of the drawbacks.

The third incredible thing is that Jen got to eat dinner off a tablecloth draped over a folding table right by the trail. That's because the Pharrs' close family friends, the Smiths—who are mentioned in Jen's book, *Becoming Odyssa*—live in Banner Elk, and they came out en masse to 19E to support Jen and feed her copious amounts of lasagna at her last road crossing of the day. Also, their youngest son Nathaniel, who ran cross-country at UNC, hiked a 10.4-mile stretch with Jen from Walnut Mountain to 19E and then he and his sister Catherine climbed another mile and a half with her toward Roan Mountain.

The fourth incredible thing is that I got to sit in a hot tub. Ok, that has nothing to do with Jen, but it sure made me happy. After she passed by 19E, she and Rambler (who is spending his last night with Jen on the trail) headed toward Doll Flats while I followed the Smiths to Catherine's and Jason's house, where the entire extended family was gathering for a big dinner.

I had a lot of fun meeting everyone, eating a delicious dinner, and then later, sitting in the hot tub while Jason and Catherine told me about how they met, what they hoped to do in the future, and how the Christmas tree industry works. (Catherine's dad works in it.) It was a great night. And an incredible day. For Jen . . . and for me.

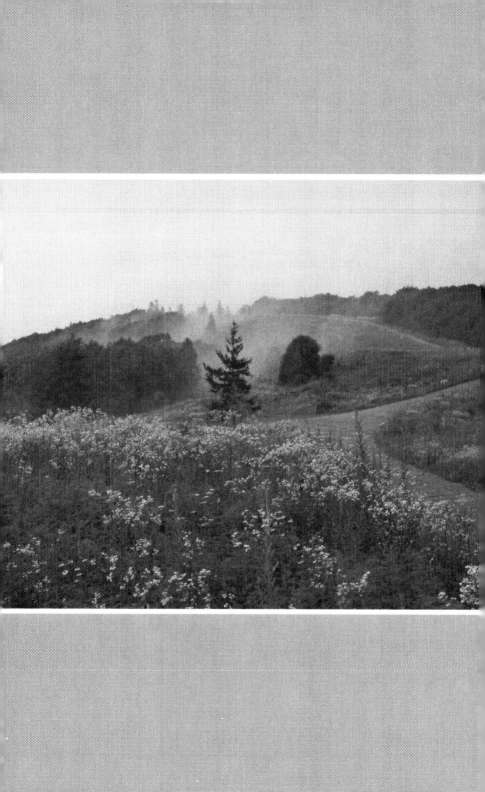

DAY 40

45.5 MILES

START TIME: 5:05 AM ✦ END TIME: 8:30 PM

Jen had another great day on the trail with lots of friends, especially young friends, coming out to support her.

She got an early start as usual and made it to Carvers Gap by 8:25 or so. Rambler, who hiked in with Jen last night, headed back toward 19E to pick up his car and drive around to meet us. After he gave us her gear, he headed north toward Pennsylvania.

I can't emphasize enough how much Rambler helped us on the trip. We may name our first child Rambler. Really. We may. I mean, my name is Brew, and I don't think the name Rambler would be much weirder than that.

Anyway, Serena Smith, her brother, Ted, and his daughter, Sophie, met us at Carvers Gap. Ted and Sophie hiked the 5.4-mile stretch to Hughes Gap with Jen. They're both tall and athletic, probably the only people Jen has hiked with who can match her stride. They arrived at Hughes Gap at 10:20 and Jen took a short break, then Sophie struck out with her again to climb Little Rock Knob before turning around.

It was neat to have Ted and Sophie hike with Jen because they had hosted Jen at their home in the Berkshires during Jen's 2005 AT thru-hike and they're mentioned in *Becoming Odyssa*.

Jen reached Iron Mountain Gap by 1:25 and was excited to meet up with some trail runner friends from Asheville: Mike Jackson and Adam Hill, as well future trail runners Asa and Annie, who are Adam's kids. Mike hiked to Beauty Spot with

Jen, and Adam and I drove around to wait for Mike's wife Renee and their kids Zoe, Zane (who was in my 6th grade class two years ago and is one of my favorite students ever), Zia, and Zella, who came out to cheer Jen on.

From there, Adam, Annie, and Asa hiked up the trail to meet Jen and Mike. As they were all coming back, the kids started racing to the cars. Jen held Asa back and yelled for Annie to run faster so she could win. They were all cracking up.

Later the youngest kids played mini tennis on the gravel road and dumped ice on each other while we drank from a Shiva IPA growler that Adam delivered from the Asheville Brewing Company. Also, Renee brought us a copy of the *New York Times* so we could see the article in print. (If you haven't seen it yet, here's the link: http://www.nytimes.com/2011/07/24/sports/speed-hiker-pharr-davis-thrives-on-rhythms-of-appalachian-trail.html).

Having the kids around made for an atypical record attempt, but Jen loved it, probably because she loves kids and because it gave her a sense of normalcy.

Mike hiked down to Indian Grave Gap with Jen and then the Jackson/Hill crew headed home while Jen got ready for the final 10.6-mile stretch to the Nolichucky River near Erwin, Tennessee.

I drove to Erwin and met our friends Jeff and Heather, their baby boy, Chase, and Heather's brother, Hampton, who's going to hike with Jen for a couple of days. We sent Hampton up the trail to meet her and then Jeff, Heather, Chase, and I had the unique and terrible experience of getting caught between TWO cargo trains. We were trapped in that purgatory for about 10 minutes. Eventually one of the trains passed and we were able to escape and get some nachos and enchiladas at a cheap Mexican restaurant.

Around 8 o'clock, we headed back to the trail to organize the car and wait for Jen and Hampton. They came down around

8:30. Jen gave Chase a big hug then carried him across the Nolichucky River toward Uncle Johnny's Hostel. For the record, Chase is probably the heaviest weight Jen has carried this entire trip.

From there we all went to the Super 8 Motel and spent a few minutes chatting while Jen ate her enchiladas and rice, then we prayed together that this last stretch would go well, that Jen would stay safe and healthy, and that the two of us would have enough energy to fight the good fight and finish the race.

I vaguely remember an early 80s sitcom called "One Day at a Time." (Jen, of course, would have no recollection of this show because she's five years younger than me. She reminds me often.) Well, that's a little too ambitious for us. For the rest of the hike, Jen's going to take it one step at a time, and I'm going to take it one road at a time. That's what we've done all along, but the strategy's becoming more and more important the closer we get to the end.

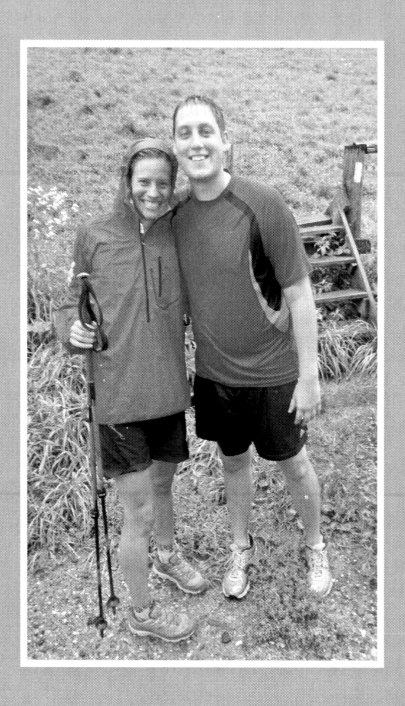

DAY 41
47.2 MILES

Today Jen had more miles, more visits, and—at long last—rain.

I dropped her off early at Uncle Johnny's Hostel and the Nolichucky River then I went back to the hotel to get some more sleep.

When Hampton and I eventually hit the road, it took us a few extra minutes to find the trail crossing at Spivey Gap. I'd like to blame it on the rain and the semi-darkness, but every once in a while, I just miss the trail. We eventually spotted it and for the first time in over 6 weeks, Jen and I were back in North Carolina. Woohoo!

After we convinced Hampton NOT to take his can of lima beans, (apparently, he has a lima bean fixation. Which is fine. I'm not judging. But on the trail, they're a bad idea because they're too heavy) the two of them struck out on a 13.4-mile stretch to Sam's Gap. They managed to avoid the rain on top of Little Bald and Big Bald, which were the only exposed sections on the trail today. So that was good.

I went back to Erwin to check e-mail, make some calls, pick up a map from Uncle Johnny's and a few other things from the grocery store. Then I made one of the best decisions of the entire trip: I stopped at the Dari Ace. (I have no idea why it's spelled that way. I meant to ask but I forgot.).

I ordered a bacon double cheeseburger for Jen and bacon cheeseburgers for Hampton and me. It took a while but, wow, were those burgers worth the wait. Next time you're in Erwin, do yourself a favor and stop by the Dari Ace.

From there, I headed down to Sam's Gap to wait for Jen and Hampton and to meet Jen's Samford friend, Mark Catlin, and our Asheville friends, Matthew and Erica Johnson, and their one-year-old, Eliza.

Matthew and Erica brought Jen homemade cookies and a milkshake from an Asheville joint called French Fryz. And Mark brought a video of his toddler son blowing Jen kisses and wishing her good luck.

Matthew and Erica hiked in with Eliza to meet Jen and Hampton. Eventually, they all came down the trail and Jen took a short break. Then Mark hiked the next 8.2 miles with her to Devils Fork Gap while Hampton and I drove the cars around and the Johnsons went to Erwin to play in the Nolichucky River.

Mark hadn't planned on hiking with Jen. He'd just driven all the way from Raleigh because he's a great guy and he wanted to encourage her. But Jen managed to rope him into hiking a stretch. Before they set out, Mark said, "I may not be able to keep up." Jen smiled and said, "That's ok. I'll drop you if you're slow."

I didn't really think she would drop him. But she did. She came plowing down a cow pasture during another rain shower without Mark. He did make it down to the car before she finished her break, so they were able to say goodbye.

Mark gushed about what a freak Jen was. I tried to make him feel better by explaining that lots of folks have had trouble keeping up with her. He told me that in college, he and another guy would say, "How far could Jen Pharr go if Jen Pharr could go far?" This afternoon, he said, "I guess she could go the length of the Appalachian Trail."

Hampton hiked the final 14 miles of the day with Jen to Camp Creek Bald. I managed to find the road and made it to the trail with her dinner as they walked up, so it was perfect timing.

We're looking forward to tomorrow when Jen will hike more miles and have more visitors. We're kind of hoping, though, that she won't have more rain.

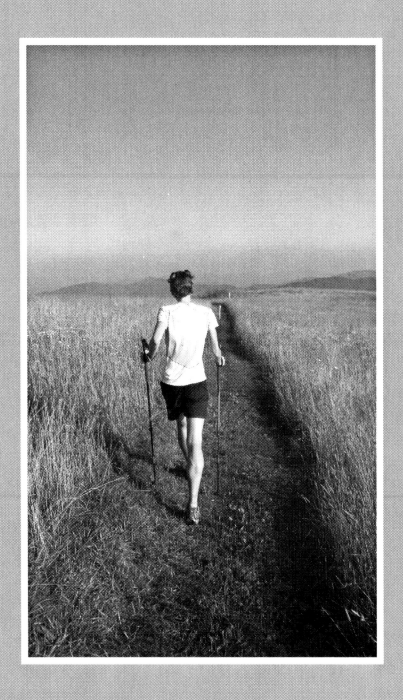

DAY 42

50.8 MILES

Today was the kind of day that separates the men from the boys—or in this case, the women from the girls.

Jen set out from Camp Creek Bald at 5:05 and reached Allen Gap a little later than expected at 7:30. It was supposed to be a 6.2-mile stretch, and Jen's been hiking consistently at about 3 mph, so what we deduced from her slightly late arrival this morning and her early arrival last night was that I met them a mile or so farther north than I'd intended.

Jen wasn't bothered by it but she did look pretty wiped out. Her best pair of custom insoles weren't dry this morning so she'd worn an older pair which made her feet hurt pretty bad.

I was a little concerned that she might not want to go all the way to Snowbird Mountain as planned. At one point, it looked like she'd have to hike until close to 11 pm to make it.

But she hiked the roughly 8-mile stretch from Allen Gap to Tanyard Gap in about two hours and twenty minutes, then she hiked the 5.9-mile stretch from Tanyard to Hot Springs in an hour and forty-five minutes.

By the time she reached Hot Springs, she had an enormous cheering section that would rival any stage on the Tour de France. Ok, maybe it wasn't *that* big, but she did have at least a dozen people rooting her on as she walked down Main Street. The crowd consisted of Heather and Chase Killebrew, Heather's in-laws Barbara and Kerry, Matthew and Eliza Johnson, Ryan and Amanda Weaver, Hampton, two of Hampton's friends from Weaverville, Mike and Jessica from the Hendersonville

Times-News, and me. She cruised down the sidewalk with the reporters then took a break to eat chicken fingers and Ben & Jerry's at the south end of town.

Matthew did a 6.6-mile stretch with her to Garenflo Gap, then Kerry offered to hike a 7.8-mile stretch with her. I was kind of skeptical that he could keep up. But I should have known better. He's retired military. He did an awesome job.

Jen hiked the final 14.2 miles of the day on her own, reaching Max Patch at 6:35 and Snowbird Mountain by 9:25.

Snowbird Mountain is not an easy access point, and I might not have made it up there unless a local kid in a camouflage pick-up hadn't offered to drive me to the base of the mountain and show me where to start climbing.

Jen dug deep today. And she'll almost certainly have to dig deep a few more times during these last 250 miles. There's no telling whether she'll set a new record or not, but she's going to give it everything she's got. That's all she can do and that's all we can hope for.

Jen enters the Smokies tomorrow. If you've read her book, you know she got struck by lightning here in 2005. Here's hoping that doesn't happen again.

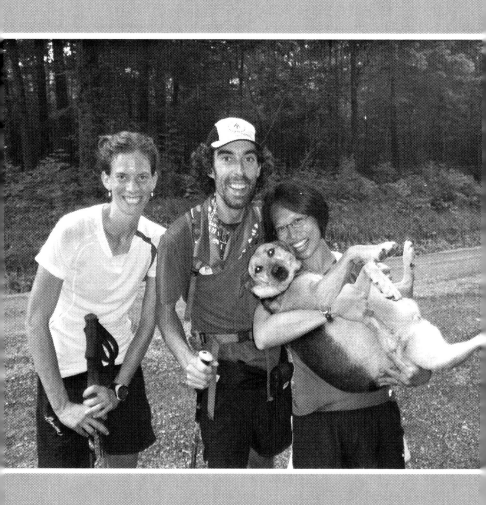

DAY 43
46.3 MILES

Well, I'm happy to report that Jen is halfway through the Smokies . . . and she has NOT been struck by lightning yet.

She woke up at the usual time and started climbing down Snowbird Mountain. And a few minutes later I had the tent and gear in the car and was heading down the mountain, too.

Several days ago, Matt-freakin'-Kirk agreed to hike with Jen again, this time through Great Smoky Mountain National Park. We were really psyched about that, but we were also concerned about the two 30+ mile stretches of trail through the park that had no road crossings. (That's Davenport Gap to Newfound Gap and Clingmans Dome to Fontana Dam).

I wanted to make those monster stretches as easy as possible for them so when a trail runner from Knoxville named Kevin Hancock contacted me on Facebook several weeks ago to offer his services, I took him up on it.

Kevin and I met at Davenport Gap around 6:25 am and I gave him food for the re-supply: a ham and cheese wrap, lots of snacks, juice water, and a Pepsi. He headed off toward Cosby at 6:45 and started hiking up the Low Gap side trail, which intersects with the AT about 14 miles into the 31.3-mile stretch from Davenport to Newfound Gap.

5 minutes after Kevin left, Matt and Lily Kirk drove up with Uhwarrie chasing them up the gravel road. He'd been running all the way from the North Carolina border. Which was only two miles away, but still.

The Kirks brought two McGriddles for Jen and two sausage

and egg biscuits for me. (I have to say, I've really grown fond of McDonald's these last six weeks. I love the sausage burritos and sweet tea on the $1 menu, the frappes that cost half as much as Starbucks, and the free wifi. Of course, we'll detox when we get home and start eating real fruits and vegetables again, but McDonald's has really come through for us since the hike began.)

Anyway, Jen reached Davenport Gap around 7:35 and she and Matt were off by 7:50. Lily headed to Joyce Kilmer with Uwharrie and I headed to that quaint little hamlet nestled at the foot of the Smokies: Gatlinburg.

The rear windows on our car have been stuck in the down position for the past several days. We were lucky it didn't rain on us and that no one snatched our laptops during that time, but we didn't want to push our luck, so I went into town to get them fixed, at least temporarily.

But that wasn't the only thing I did during my roughly eight hours of free time. I've been hearing for years about Pigeon Forge, and I wanted to see what all the fuss was about. It's kind of like Myrtle Beach. Or Vegas. Except Vegas has glittering casinos and five star restaurants, and Pigeon Forge has pancake joints and putt-putt.

Speaking of putt-putt, I played a round at one of the most prestigious putt-putt courses in North America. Since I'm into comparisons in this blog, I think I would say it's the Pebble Beach of putt-putt: open to the public, but very exclusive. It's called Hillbilly Golf. It costs $11 per round (not cheap by putt-putt standards) and it's on the side of a ridge so you have to ride an incline rail to get to the course. I played there on a family reunion over 25 years ago. And it was better than I remembered.

I had a makeable hole-in-one on number 18 to make even par for the round, but I choked. Ugh. I was really hoping for a Tiger Woods moment: not the "cheating on your wife with a dozen women" type of moment, but the "winning the U.S. Open with a torn ACL" type of moment.

After putt-putt, I headed toward Newfound Gap where I rendezvoused with our pastor John Greene and our friend Isaiah Mosteller. John loves hiking and is uber-supportive of Jen's record attempt. Every Sunday before church, I call to give him an update and ask for prayers during the service.

Isaiah loves hiking, too, and was more than happy to handle the re-supply between Clingman's and Fontana Dam on day two of the Smokies. So he'd come out early to spend the night with us.

Jen and Matt reached Newfound Gap around 6:25. They took a 20-minute pit stop then continued climbing toward Clingmans. We met them a couple times along the road before the final stop under the Observation Tower.

All in all, it was another solid day for Jen and the Pit Crew. We were thankful to have good weather and to have reached Clingmans Dome, which is the highest point on the AT. (That's right, New Englanders. It's higher than your blessed Mt. Washington.) I wish very much that I could say "It's all downhill from here," but we all know these last 200 miles will be brutal.

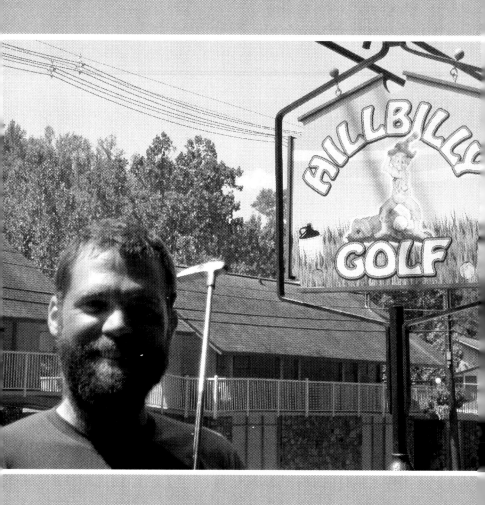

DAY 44
48.2 MILES

START TIME: 5:05 AM   ✦   END TIME: 9:10 PM

Jen got a good night's sleep and was back on the trail before dawn again, and Matt Kirk was out there with her.

One of our strategies this trip—and there are a lot of them—has been for Jen to be hiking by 5 or so every morning. It's taken a lot of discipline but an extra hour or two on the trail every day means an extra 3-6 miles, and that makes a huge difference.

Isaiah and I made our way over to Cades Cove where we parked his car at the Anthony Creek trailhead and drove back to the Low Gap trailhead. Isaiah hiked from there to the Bote Mountain trail, then headed east toward the AT where he met up with Jen and Matt at the trail junction for a re-supply.

He hiked with them for three miles before heading down the Russell Field trail then the Anthony Creek trail to his car. While Isaiah was hiking with Jen and Matt, he recited "Isaiah 40," which he'd memorized for his 40th birthday when he hiked 40 miles from the French Broad River up to Black Balsam near Asheville. The two most meaningful verses in that chapter to Isaiah—and I would say, Jen, too—are the last two, which say, "Even youths grow tired and weary, and young men stumble and fall; but those who hope in the Lord will renew their strength. They will soar on wings like eagles; they will run and not grow weary, they will walk and not be faint." Jen's been worn out a lot but I would never describe her as weak or "faint," and we attribute that to having faith that God would sustain and strengthen her.

She and Matt reached the southern end of the Smokies at Fontana Dam around 3:40. Lily and Uwharrie were there to greet them and so was Jen's dad, Yorke, who'd come out mid-day and is planning to stay with us until the end. Our photographer friend Maureen came out, too, to document the last 165 miles.

There were also a couple of well-wishers at the dam: a hiker named Tom who'd retired to the Knoxville area from Long Island and a Fontana Dam volunteer from Chattanooga.

Isaiah came to the dam, too, on his way home from Cades Cove. He and Matt returned some of our gear then they, Lily and Uwharrie headed home, Isaiah to Asheville, and the Kirks to Marion.

Jen hiked the remaining 15.8 miles by herself. We met her at Yellow Creek Gap a little before 7 pm, then Yorke went into Robbinsville to pick up dinner from the Carolina Kitchen Smokehouse and get our rooms situated at the Two Wheel Inn, which is a sweet little hotel that caters mostly to bikers who come out to ride the Tail of the Dragon on the southern end of Smokies. The hotel was clean and had small garages for the motorcycles, which of course was useless to us but was still cool.

Jen got to shower for the first time in four days and eat a BBQ sandwich and onion rings for dinner. She's in great spirits and is ready for the final 150 miles. We're hoping to see a big crowd on Springer in the coming days.

animal sightings: Jen and Matt trailed a black bear for a hundred yards or so this morning. Jen said he kept looking back at them like he was thinking, "Why are you guys following me? Why can't you just leave me alone?"

Also, when Isaiah and I drove around to Cades Cove this morning, I saw a toddler fox run across the road then stand and stare at me in the tall grass. He was pretty darn cute.

And to put things in perspective . . . If Jen had stopped at

Fontana Dam this afternoon, and hiked only 12 miles a day for the next 13.75 days, she *still* would be able to break her 2008 women's record of 57 days, 8 hours, 13 minutes.

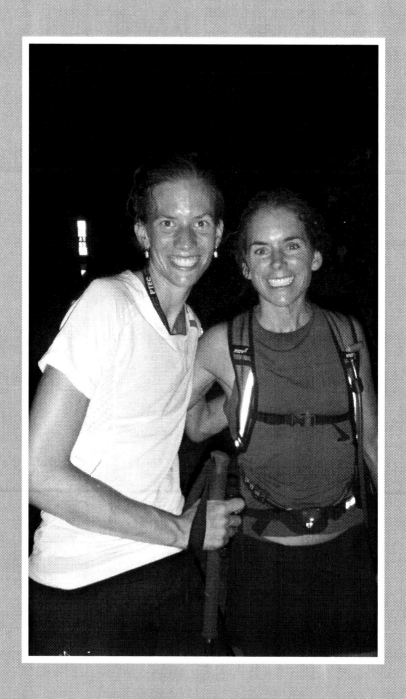

DAY 45
52.2 MILES

START TIME: 5:05 AM ✦ END TIME: 10:20 PM

Jen drew 52 miles closer to Springer today over some really difficult terrain.

I drove her out to Stecoah Gap at 4:45 am and she was hiking by 5. She reached the Nantahala Outdoor Center by 9:25, and was greeted there by Tiffany Shuler of Sylva and her 4-year-old daughter Makalyn. They've heard Jen speak two or three times throughout western North Carolina and have become friends and fans. Makalyn brought Jen an AT picture book that she'd made. She spent most of the time splashing in the river while Tiffany chatted with Jen and took photos.

Anne Lundblad, who's an accomplished trail runner from Asheville, also met Jen at the NOC. She was excited to keep Jen company all day, and she did a fantastic job, hiking over 40 miles with her and carrying her snacks and juice water.

Jen and Anne had a really difficult 7.9-mile climb to Tellico Gap out of the Nantahala Gorge that they completed in only two hours and fifteen minutes. From there, they headed to Burningtown Gap and then on to Wayah Bald. They made the tower by 3:24. I was hoping to get some pictures of Jen at the summit, but I spent most of the pit stop looking for my cell phone, which had fallen out of my pocket at Burningtown Gap. Yorke offered to drive all the way back to look for it. It probably took him 45 minutes to get back there, and he found it right before it started raining.

From Wayah Bald, Jen and Anne got to Wayah Gap in a little over an hour. Yorke went into Franklin to find a hotel and pick up some chicken fingers at Zaxby's. Mo and I also made a quick trip into town to check e-mail and pick up a USB card reader from Kmart.

The girls arrived at Winding Stair Gap (U.S. 64) at 6:20 and were back on the trail by 6:35. 3.7 miles later, they reached Rock Gap and pressed on so they could make it over the really difficult stretch around Albert Mountain and get into Mooney Gap as early as possible.

They reached it at 10:20. After a couple of photos and hugs, Anne caught a ride back to the NOC with Yorke, and Jen ate the rest of her chicken fingers.

About 10 seconds after Yorke and Anne left, Carl Laniak pulled up in his blue minivan. Carl is a trail runner from Athens, Georgia. We're psyched that he's going to hike the last 96.4 miles with Jen. And 76.4 of those miles are in North Georgia, which Carl knows like the back of his hand.

We're still hoping that Jen will reach Springer by 5:30 pm on Sunday afternoon. On the second to last day of her 2008 record attempt, she hiked 65.4 miles. And because her goal has always been to do her best (not necessarily to break the record), she's decided that she wants to do something similar tomorrow.

We're going to watch her really closely to make sure she's not at risk in any way. But this is Jen's hike and she knows what she can and can't do. We're hoping that she stays healthy and safe these final two days and that we all make the right decisions.

car update: The exterior of the car got four de facto baths in 30 hours from the rain showers and thunderstorms between Damascus and 19E. But we've had warm, sunny days since then and we've driven on lots of dirt roads so the Highlander has taken on that Manny Ramirez helmet look again.

As for the interior, it started emitting a ripe, pungent aroma just before we entered the Smokies. And it was really bizarre because it practically happened overnight. I think maybe one of Jen's wet outfits got shoved under a seat or something. I could look for it, but I'm too tired to care.

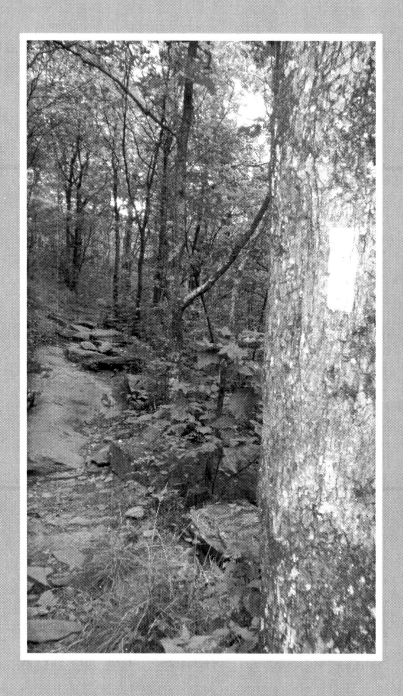

DAY 46
60.2 MILES

START TIME: 3:05 AM   ✦   END TIME: 10:40 PM

Be forewarned: Day 46 was epic, and the blog entry is longer than usual, which is saying something because these entries seem to be getting longer and longer. Sorry for that.

For the second time on an AT record attempt, Jen completed a 60-mile day.

Jen (and therefore we . . . ugh) woke up at 2:45 am. When Carl climbed out of his minivan, I said, "Good morning." Then I started wondering if 2:45 counted as "morning" or not. I decided it depends on whether you've just woken up or haven't gone to bed yet. So for us, it was morning.

They started hiking a little after 3 am. Mo and I tried to get a little more sleep. I don't know how it was for Mo, but I had a pretty tough time. I was too worried that—in the dark, as fatigued as she was—Jen was going to wipe out or twist her ankle or do something else that would jeopardize the hike in the last hundred miles.

But they arrived at Deep Gap without incident at 7:30, a little later than expected but I was happy for that because it meant they took their time.

From Deep Gap they had 15.8 miles to Dicks Creek Gap. Mo and I had some time to kill so we drove into Hiawassee to check e-mail and find some meds for my poison ivy. I must have gotten it using the men's tree (Rambler's term, not mine) in Cades Cove. It's the worst poison ivy I've ever had because it's right on the back of my knee where it stays sweaty. It also doesn't help that I haven't showered in a few days. One blister looks like a cinnamon flavored Jelly Belly. (Sorry. Was that too graphic? I think we established with the pregnancy test blog and the "flat and fast" small boobs blog that this would be a mostly unfiltered journal.)

Anyway, now I have a torn ACL on my right knee and a gnarly rash on my left, which all makes for some interesting walking.

We got to Dicks Creek Gap around 11:50. Jen and Carl (I haven't mentioned this yet, but the obvious nickname for him—given that his last name is Laniak and that, among other things, he's completed 70+ miles at the Barkley [a 100-miler in TN that only 10 people have finished in 25 years]—is Laniak the Maniac) cruised in around 12:25. They'd definitely picked up the pace a bit from the last stretch so I was starting to feel better that Jen would have a chance to complete a 60+ mile day and still get in at a reasonable time.

They didn't stay long but before they left, I asked Carl if there was another access point between Dicks Creek and Tray Gaps. He said we could drive toward Addis Gap (5.4 miles south of Dicks Creek) and then hike the last ½ mile from there. I've been trying to meet Jen at every possible road crossing so I decided we'd give it a go. Also, we owed Jen a milkshake because we forgot to bring her one at Dicks Creek. Also, I like hiking in—you could almost say I *need* it—since I can't do any real hiking on the AT this summer and it helps me feel more connected to Jen and what she's doing.

So the Pit Crew drove back to Hiawassee to pick up a last major round of groceries at Ingles and a chocolate shake at the Dairy Queen, then we headed toward Addis Gap.

When I'd driven as far as I could, I jumped out of the car and headed up the trail. I'd been hiking for about a ½ mile and still wasn't anywhere near the gap when I turned a corner on the gravel road and had my best animal encounter of the summer.

About 25 feet in front of me, a beautiful, medium sized grey-and-white peppered screech owl (I had to Google that) was cleaning himself in the middle of the road. I froze and he went about his business for another five or ten seconds; then he must have realized somebody was watching him because he swiveled his head slightly. Then a couple seconds later he swiveled his head all the way around so he could see me.

He stared at me and I stared back. Then he turned his whole body, took a couple of steps, flapped his wings, and started flying low and right at me. I had Jen's blue pit stop chair over my left shoulder and was about to bring it around to cover myself, but then when he was about ten feet away, he pulled up and off to the left and found the nearest branch. We stared at each other for another minute or two. Then he sort of lost interest and started cleaning himself again.

It was an awesome moment and probably the only thing that could have distracted me from hiking up to meet Jen and Carl.

I reached Addis Gap a few minutes after 2 pm and was beginning to worry I'd miss them, but they strolled in ten minutes later. Jen inhaled the milkshake and Carl told me he was glad I was there because he was pretty wiped out and was hoping to take a break for a stretch or two so he could night hike at the end of the day. When she finished her milkshake, she took the pack and kept walking and Carl and I headed down to the car.

We drove around to Tray Gap with Maureen. (Yorke had met us at Dicks Creek Gap then headed to Amicalola Falls State Park to pick up Jen's older brother Jones. The two of them drove back to Mooney Gap to pick up Carl's minivan and bring it around to where we'd finish so Carl could have his normal sleeping arrangement for the night.)

The drive to Tray Gap took a long time but as we pulled up, we got to see a young black bear foraging down a side trail. He watched us for a while then sauntered off into the underbrush and resurfaced a few minutes later for some more photo ops. He was probably 40 yards away. I was happy to have a couple of animal encounters today since Jen's had so many throughout the hike.

She didn't stop long at Tray Gap before heading on to Indian Grave Gap. There have been only two times on the trail where I've told people who Jen was and what she was doing. Both times involved groups of young girls, and Indian Grave Gap was the second time.

This particular group of teenagers was on a wilderness therapy hike. I told them that my wife would be coming down the trail in a few minutes and that she was trying to break the overall record on the Appalachian Trail and that it's always been held by men. Ever the educator, I guess I saw it as a teachable moment.

Anyway, the girls cheered her on and yelled "Girl power!" and "You go, girl!" as she walked through. Jen gave me a dirty look because she's shy and doesn't like attention, which seems counterintuitive given her predilection for public speaking, but she's a total introvert and recharges by being by herself or with me.

From Indian Grave Gap, she had only 2.6 miles to Unicoi Gap. She got there around 5:20 and left with Carl around 5:35 for the last major stretch of the day, a 13.8-miler to Hogpen Gap.

Mo and I drove from Unicoi Gap into Helen to get some Mexican food, a few more groceries, and a map of North Georgia. (I had AT maps but they didn't include all of the roads we needed to use on the final day.)

Helen was a little overwhelming. I think it's referred to as "Georgia's Gatlinburg." It's nowhere near as shocking as the real Gatlinburg or Pigeon Forge, but since we had to walk down the crowded sidewalks and get stuck in some weekend traffic, it felt worse.

I was hoping we could meet up with my parents, who were supposed to arrive in Helen this evening. But they got stuck in Atlanta traffic (imagine that) and didn't make it in time.

On our way out of town, Mo and I coordinated with Yorke and Jones so they'd know where to bring Carl's car. They'd been driving for hours and they really wanted to get back to the lodge at Amicalola, but they made the extra effort to track us down so Carl could sleep in his van, and I really appreciated that.

We got to Hogpen Gap around 9:15. I made some phone calls to tell our friends and family when they should arrive at Springer then headed down to Tesnatee Gap to set up the tent while Mo stayed at Hogpen to wait for Jen and Carl. I got back up about 10:15, twenty minutes or so before they came through. It was an incredible thing to see those headlamps bobbing down the trail toward us. Mo and I started whooping and yelling, and I cranked "The Cave" by Mumford & Sons. They'd finished 59.3 miles but Jen wanted to have a 60-mile day, a "statement day," as Warren calls it. Carl dropped the pack and they crossed the road and headed up one final short climb before descending to Tesnatee, .9 miles away.

When they got down there, I yelled, "60 *freaking* miles!" Jen pretty much collapsed in my arms as she came out of the woods, as much out of satisfaction and pleasure, I think, as out of exhaustion.

We had their Mexican food waiting for them. I had a Highland Oatmeal Porter for Carl and Wet Ones for Jen. Carl poured a gallon of water over his head in lieu of a shower. Jen doctored her feet for a few minutes then set the alarm for 2:45 again. I cried a few tears. Ok, not really, but I was *not* happy about waking up at 2:45 for a second consecutive "morning." Then we hit the sack, knowing that Jen needed to do "only" 36.2 miles tomorrow to have a new overall AT record.

One other funny thing I forgot to mention: I asked Mo to get me a small Heath Bar Blizzard from Dairy Queen when we'd gone back to Hiawassee. I grabbed it from her when we pulled off GA 75 and started eating it on the way up to Addis Gap. I'd eaten about half of it before it was time to start hiking up toward the trail. You can imagine my surprise and displeasure when Carl and I got back to the car and I saw my month-old phone (my first new one in almost 7 years) partially submerged in my half eaten Blizzard.

It had fallen out of my pocket while I was driving. I tried to drain it and clean it off, but I could tell it was a lost cause when I saw the frothy remnants dripping from behind the keypad. The day before, I'd been really frustrated when I left my phone at Burningtown Gap. But this time, all I could do was laugh. With the 30-40 calls and the dozen or so texts I'd been receiving every day for the past week, I couldn't decide whether the timing was terrible . . . or perfect.

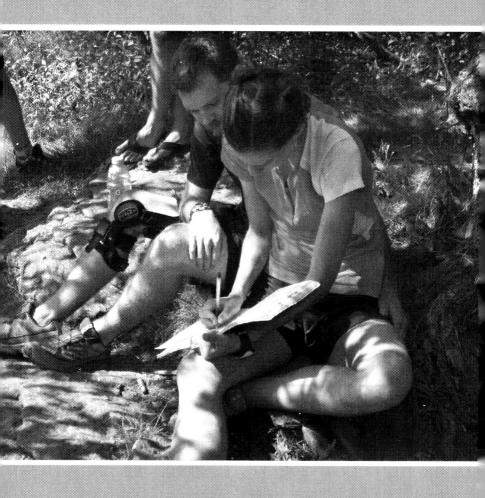

DAY 47
(AKA, DAY THE LAST)
36.2 MILES

START TIME: 2:45 AM ✦ END TIME: 3:26 PM

Jen, Carl, Maureen, and I woke up at 2:45 again. Jen was making some terrible sounds as she got ready. Like, "I've been hiking 47 miles a day for 45 days straight and have gotten a total of 7.5 hours of sleep the last two nights" sort of sounds.

Carl said, "This is how it feels." We talked later about that and what he meant—more or less—was, "This is how it feels when you've pushed yourself to the limit. And this is what you've got to overcome if you're going to do something great." I thought I knew what he meant when he said it. But I could tell Jen didn't because she just groaned some more.

Anyway, they set off at 3:05. I was nervous again because you never know what can happen when someone's night hiking on less than 4 hours of sleep. But Jen and Carl reached Neels Gap around 5:25.

Neither of them touched the hard boiled egg and mozzarella string cheese wraps I'd made them. I have to admit, I was a little insulted. I've been getting rave reviews for my wraps all trip—beginning with Dutch—and I'm not used to being rejected.

Carl chugged two Ensure shakes then they began climbing Blood Mountain a few minutes later. Maureen and I drove around to Woody Gap. When we got there at 6:05, Jen's two brothers, Jones and James, were there. (Jones and his wife Jackie flew down from New York by way of Charlotte, where they have a place. James, Lindsay, and Hazel came straight from Litchfield Beach in South Carolina.)

I asked them if they knew Jen wouldn't be there until 9, and they said yes. James added, "This [waking up ridiculously early] is what I get for hanging out with my brother the banker."

We talked until 7 or so then I told them I needed to take a nap. James took a nap, too. I think Jones stayed awake and talked to Maureen, but I'm not sure because I was drooling on my headrest for the next hour and a half.

Jen came in at 9:05, but Carl was nowhere in sight. She told us he had to stop early in the 10.6-mile stretch because he'd gotten sick. Carl had been having stomach issues for weeks. Plus, he'd just finished helping organize a road race that ran through Tennessee from Missouri to Georgia.

Jen said she waited for him for a few minutes, then decided she couldn't control when he got to her but she could control when she got to us. I should mention that, like any good Sherpa, Carl was carrying the snacks and drinks.

So after Jen got down a Pepsi—along with one of my gourmet and underappreciated egg wraps—she elaborated on how she'd felt with no food or water for 10+ miles. At one point, she said half-jokingly, "I saw a lot of animals on that stretch—I just don't know if they were all real."

But she felt better after taking in more snacks and juice water, and she and Jones were heading for Gooch Gap by 9:15. Maureen and I drove around while James waited for Carl to come out of the woods.

Apparently, Jones was really pushing Jen and saying things like, "Come on . . . you should be running this! This is a runnable section." So she ran for a while and they got in at 10:21. James and Carl were nowhere in sight so Jones hiked/ran the next section to Cooper Gap.

At some point along the way, I stopped to check the map and realized that James and Carl were behind Maureen's enormous diesel engine Ford truck. When we got to Cooper Gap, Carl told us how he'd stopped so Jen couldn't hear him throw up because she said if she'd heard him, she'd have probably gotten sick, too. So he was sprawled out on all fours in the middle of the trail, puking his guts out for five minutes.

Eventually, he got to his feet and started running down Blood Mountain to catch up with Jen, but he jostled his stomach enough that he got sick again. Then he realized he wasn't going to catch her, so he took a side trail down to Lake Winfield Scott Recreation Area where he hoped to hitch a ride to Woody Gap.

A guy in a truck took Carl a mile or two before he had to turn off, but no one else would pick him up so he had to road walk the remaining 7 miles. But he made it. And we were glad. The Pit Crew had gone 46 days without a lost-time injury. We didn't want to ruin the streak so close to the end.

Jen and Jones reached Cooper Gap around 11:35, and James hiked with her from there.

Eventually, people realized that they couldn't reach me on my phone because I'd thrown it in a Dairy Queen Blizzard so they started tracking me down on Jen's phone. It turned out to be a good thing because I was able to give my parents directions to Hightower Gap and they were able to meet us there.

Jen and James came through around 12:45 and only stayed for a few minutes before pressing on toward Three Forks, which was 4 miles away. At this point, Jen could definitely smell the barn. (If you're not familiar with that expression, it's referring to the way a donkey or mule in the field speeds up at the end of the day because it knows that the sooner it's done, the sooner it can get back to the stall and rest. Trail runners do the same thing. And no, I don't normally compare my wife to a beast of burden.)

My sister Dearing and I drove around to Three Forks where Warren was waiting. He'd rearranged his schedule and driven hours out of his way so he could hand her a cup of water from the stream.

When Jen got there, I cranked John Cowan's version of "Mighty Clouds of Joy" from the Telluride Bluegrass Festival compilation. (She asked me to sing that whenever I walked with her this summer on the flat stretches of trail.)

From Three Forks, Jen and James had 3.3 miles to Forest Service Road 42. They reached it around 3:05. Everyone was on top of Springer except Jen's mom—who was waiting to take photos of Jen and James—and me. I played "The Cave" by Mumford & Sons. That's been the unofficial theme song this summer because it talks about "strength through pain" and it makes lots of allusions to the Odyssey.

Jen started sobbing. I cried, too. We hugged, and I said, "You did it . . ." And she said, "No. *We* did it . . ." We held hands on our way up Springer. I asked if she would want to hug people or take photos or do anything else before finishing, and she said, "I just want to touch the rock."

I asked her if she wanted to know who was here and she said "no." Every now and then, she would take gasping breaths and start crying, but then she'd regain her composure.

Jen's family friend Serena, who'd fed her lasagna on a table-cloth in northeast Tennessee, took some photos a hundred yards or so from the rock. When we got near the summit, we could hear all the people.

We came out of the woods onto the granite slab and everyone had their cameras out. There were about 45 people there. They all started cheering and taking photos. Jen started crying again. We touched the sign together then we hugged and cried some more. It was kind of funny having so many people around. Everyone recognized how awkward it was and as the cameras flashed someone said something about a *"private* moment." Everyone laughed.

Jen looked at her watch to mark the time. 3:26 pm. 46 days, 11 hours, and 20 minutes after she touched the sign on Katahdin. Then we sat on the rock and took it all in.

Jen saw her Samford friend Emily who'd driven all the way from Mississippi with her husband Jeff. She didn't know Emily was coming so she started crying all over again. And that happened several more times because people Jen cared about so much had driven so far.

Her Samford roommate Katie had driven from Birmingham with her husband David, son Peter, and mom Beth. Mark Catlin, another Samford friend, had driven 15 hours round trip from Raleigh with his wife and son to spend an hour on top of Springer. And loads of friends, family, and strangers had travelled from western North Carolina, Tennessee, Georgia, Alabama, and South Carolina.

Warren stood off to the side taking it all in, wearing a green shirt with a white blaze on it, looking very much like a *part* of the AT. I hugged him and said "thank you." We both started to cry and he said, "thank *you* . . . thank *you* . . ." He hugged me so tight I almost couldn't breathe.

It was all very special and wonderful. Like a wedding.

After all the photos and hugs, Jen signed the register. It was short and sweet. She wrote, "Full of love, appreciation, memories, and no regrets! —Jennifer Pharr Davis "Odyssa" July 31st, 2011." Eventually people started straggling back down the mountain.

A few friends and family got lost on the way to Springer, but we got to see them in the parking lot. Jen's friend Alice, who drove up from Atlanta, brought champagne and plastic cups. We cranked Mumford & Sons again. Jen and I danced to "The Cave." After another 20 or 30 minutes, everyone said their goodbyes and we went our separate ways.

As Jen and I were driving back down Forest Service Road 42,

we stopped to ask a group of soldiers who were doing military exercises which way was the quickest down to Dahlonega. They asked if we'd been to Springer to see the endurance hiker, and we told them Jen *was* the endurance hiker. They called their sergeant over because he wanted to shake her hand and congratulate her. We thanked them for serving our country then drove toward Helen where we spent the night with our friends Frank and Lauren at Lauren's parents' mountain house.

We visited with them for a while, ate some pizza, and then went to bed. And that was the end of our arduous, sublime adventure.

PSALM 91

1 Whoever dwells in the shelter of the Most High
will rest in the shadow of the Almighty.
2 I will say of the LORD, "He is my refuge and my fortress,
my God, in whom I trust."
3 Surely he will save you
from the fowler's snare
and from the deadly pestilence.
4 He will cover you with his feathers,
and under his wings you will find refuge;
his faithfulness will be your shield and rampart.
5 You will not fear the terror of night,
nor the arrow that flies by day,
6 nor the pestilence that stalks in the darkness,
nor the plague that destroys at midday.
7 A thousand may fall at your side,
ten thousand at your right hand,
but it will not come near you.
8 You will only observe with your eyes
and see the punishment of the wicked.

9 If you say, "The LORD is my refuge,"
and you make the Most High your dwelling,
10 no harm will overtake you,
no disaster will come near your tent.
11 For he will command his angels concerning you
to guard you in all your ways;
12 they will lift you up in their hands,
so that you will not strike your foot against a stone.
13 You will tread on the lion and the cobra;
you will trample the great lion and the serpent.
14 "Because he loves me," says the LORD, "I will rescue him;
I will protect him, for he acknowledges my name.
15 He will call on me, and I will answer him;
I will be with him in trouble,
I will deliver him and honor him.
16 With long life I will satisfy him
and show him my salvation."

DAY 48
(AKA, THE 19TH HOLE)

START TIME: 12:01 AM　✦　END TIME: NEVER

I'm sitting on the porch at our friends' mountain house outside of Helen, Georgia, drinking 12-year Glenfiddich, checking e-mails, and gazing at some beautiful North Georgia mountains.

Also, I'm wearing deodorant for the first time in 46 days.

Here's a brief rundown of the past few hours: Jen slept from 10 PM to 8 AM then again from 11:30 to 2:30. Since then, she's been talking to reporters and checking www.people.com. (Three great quotes: when she first looked on the website, she said, "I missed you, *People!*" Then she said, "Tell everyone that it's important for me to catch up on hard news." And a few minutes later when she was a few pages in she said, "Oh, Kate [Catherine Middleton, Duchess of Cambridge] . . . you've done *so much* while I was on the trail.")

Also, Jen's been doing nothing. Literally. Before her late morning nap, I said, "Do you want to watch some television? Or do you want to read a magazine?" And she said, "No. I'll just sit here."

She also said she feels like she was hit by a semi-truck. But she's in good spirits—as evidenced by all her funny quotes—and she's enjoying the recovery process so far.

Tonight, we're going to eat leftover pizza, drink red wine, and watch TV. (Another great quote: Jen said earlier, "Yeah, I timed my finish so I could watch the season finale of *The Bachelorette*." She is a big fan of JP. And if I'm being honest, so am I.)

In the coming days, we'll be spending time with family

then heading to the Outdoor Retailer show in Salt Lake City before spending more time with family and returning to Asheville.

And from there, life will go on.

But before that, we want to leave you with two final thoughts. The first is this: words fall short of expressing how grateful we are for all the support we've received.

There is no way we could have accomplished this goal without the help of the entire Pit Crew, the trail visits from friends and family—especially at Springer—and the support and prayers so many people offered from afar.

And the second thought comes not from us, but from the One who "was and is and is to come" . . .

"Jesus looked at them and said, 'With man this is impossible, but with God all things are possible.'" (Matthew 19:26)

To God be the Glory.

— BREW AND JEN
(August 1, 2011)

REFLECTIONS

I t has been almost three weeks now since we finished the trail and in some ways it is all starting to feel like a dream. Brew and I returned home this past Sunday, and he started back to work today. Our house is the same, our friends are the same—if not more wonderful—and our little niece has a few more tricks, but she is still just as adorable and beautiful as when we left in June. If it were not for the peeling callus on my big toe, the tenderness in the bottom of my feet, and the blinding light-headedness that comes when I stand up, I would rarely be reminded of our record attempt this summer. And I think that's a good thing.

If I expected the trail this summer to fill a void, then I would be highly disappointed. The truth is, as wonderful as the trail is, it cannot complete you. However, it can change you. And that is why we go, each summer, and most free days and weekends during the year. The trail has helped me to become more self-confident, patient, and accepting. This summer, the trail taught me to live in the moment, appreciate the small things, and never lose sight of hope.

Most people look at our 2011 journey as an athletic feat; however, I consider it to be a love story. I love the trail, and far more than that, I love my husband. Beyond romance, I believe true love is best demonstrated through endurance and perseverance. That is what got me through the bad weather, intense pain, and many hardships this summer—a devotion to the trail and a complete trust and shared intimacy with my husband. Contrary to some reports, I have yet to receive any financial endorsements, movie deals, or lump sums since the trail, but that is not to say that I haven't been rewarded. My post-trail trophies are the e-mails and letters I received from strangers saying that our journey has encouraged them to get outside, enjoy nature, and discover their own path. My increase in wealth can be measured in memories and self-growth. And my most cherished prize is the look that I share with my husband that says, "We did it. Despite the people who told us we couldn't and against all odds, we believed in one another and we accomplished something amazing." That look, in itself, is invaluable; and it is something that no one will ever be able to take away from us.

Looking ahead, I can't wait until my body feels rested enough to return to the trail. I doubt that, for us, there will ever be a hike that compares to the intensity of this summer. Yet, I know that there will be lots of day hiking, trail runs, and long-distance backpacking trips in our future. I look forward to seeing other people go after our record on the Appalachian Trail, partly because I want them to know how much it hurts, and I also look forward to seeing the limits of human potential stretched even farther.

I believe that record holders never stand alone, they simply crawl onto the shoulders of the people who went before them. I could never have hiked the trail in 46 days if it hadn't been for the example and inspiration of Andrew Thompson. His 47-day hike is phenomenal, and I would love it if he wanted to go after the record again—after all, his initials are A.T.

Regardless of who goes after the record in the future, I am sure he or she will do it differently because of our example this summer. I doubt that record setter will spend every night at the roadside, perhaps he or she won't run, and that person will most certainly want to duplicate the support of the Pit Crew. I would love it if another woman wanted to go after the record. However, honestly, the attempt this summer was never about beating the boys. It was about doing my best—and I believed that my best was good enough for the overall record. In fact, I could have never been successful this summer without the help of the men in my life. (Thanks, guys.)

Benton MacKaye, the founder of the Appalachian Trail, believed that the purpose of long-distance trails is, "To walk. To see. To see what you see." I feel the same way. But personally, that expression has evolved in its meaning. At first it was about seeing nature, then it was about seeing nature and my true self. The words now also inspire me to see and seek out my full potential and the full potential of the trail.

I believe that people will not protect the trail unless they can see what is in front of them. And to truly see the trail involves more than just hiking. You have to be able to experience the trail, on your own terms, and in your own language. I am so thankful that the trail is there for everyone at every stage of life. It can be experienced slow or fast, in short day-hikes or long sections. As members of the trail community, it is our responsibility to overlook preferences of speed, distance, and gear. And, instead, work together to promote and protect the trail and recognize our common bond, which includes a love of nature and the belief that something powerful and positive comes from physically moving through the wilderness.

Rest assured, the next person to set the overall record on the Appalachian Trail will most certainly have pure motives and a strong love of nature. The task is too difficult otherwise.

JENNIFER PHARR DAVIS
August 2011

ACKNOWLEDGMENTS

Normally, this is the place where the author thanks those who made the book possible. But in this case, I need to start by thanking the people who made the hike possible, because without it there would be no book.

A verse in the Bible says, "Therefore, since we are surrounded by such a great cloud of witnesses, let us throw off everything that hinders and the sin that so easily entangles, and let us run with perseverance the race marked out for us." (Hebrews 12:1) Well, Jen wasn't running a race, but she certainly wouldn't have been able to complete the hike without the support of so many this summer.

First and foremost, thanks to the Pit Crew: Warren, Melissa, Steve, Rambler, Dutch, Horton, Rebecca, Doug, Matt, Lily, Uwharrie, James, Lindsay, Hazel, Mo, Serena, Catherine, Nate, Ted, Sophie, Mike, Jeff, Heather, Chase, Hampton, Mark, MJ, Kerri, Kevin, Isaiah, Yorke, Anne, Carl, and Jones.

We received constant encouragement from friends and family who came to the trail to cheer Jen on. Thanks to Eric, Gratton, the extended Smith family, Adam, Asa, Annie, Renee, Zoe, Zane, Zia, and Zella, Erica, Eliza, Barbara, Ryan, Amanda, John, Tiffany, and Makalyn.

Certain people opened their homes or helped us unexpectedly and it made our lives much easier. For their kindness and hospitality, I want to thank Bear and Honey, Adam, Kadra, Mary Ellen, Ryan, Jason, Catherine, Don, and Genevieve.

And I appreciate everyone who made the effort to be with us on Springer Mountain: Katie, David, Peter, Beth, Emily, Jeff, Frank, Lauren, Sarah, Genevieve, Louisa, Kimberly, Sam, Houck, Hank, Robbie, Dearing, Barbara, and Jackie.

The Appalachian Trail is long and winding. It climbs some of the tallest mountains in the East and traverses boulder fields that bring hikers to their knees. It's an arduous journey and a metaphor for life. Jen's family and mine have been encouraged us every step of the way, and for that I am grateful.

Now, for the book . . . Thanks to everyone in the Beaufort and Midpoint offices who have worked so vigorously to get this book on the shelf. We are fortunate to work with such a supportive company. Two people who have been especially supportive are Eric Kampmann and Margot Atwell. Eric, Beaufort's owner, met Jen at a trail conference in 2009, and he's had faith in her ever since. I am thankful to him for giving her a chance, and now for giving me a chance. I am also thankful to Margot, Beaufort's editor, who has embraced Jen's project and mine with energy and optimism. Eric and Margot have been our advocates, and they have become our friends.

Thanks to my wife, Jen. She was my reason for being on the trail, and she is my reason for being in life. I thank God continually that she is my wife and my best friend.

And finally, thanks to God for being God—the Lover of ragamuffins, the Restorer of souls. Gloria, in excelsis Deo.

"SHELTER ME" (BUDDY AND JULIE MILLER)

The earth can shake the sky come down
the mountains all fall to the ground
but I will fear none of these things
shelter me Lord underneath your wings
Dark waters rise and thunders pound
the wheels of war are going round
and all the walls are crumbling
shelter me Lord underneath your wings

Hide me underneath your wings
hide me deep inside your heart
in your refuge—cover me
the world can shake
but Lord I'm making you my hiding place

The wind can blow the rain can pour
the deluge breaks the tempest roars
but in the storm my spirit sings
when you shelter me Lord underneath your wings

Shelter me Lord
hide me underneath your wings
hide me deep inside your heart
in your refuge—cover me
the world can shake
but Lord I'm making you my hiding place

Now on the day you call for me
someday when time—no more shall be
I'll say oh death where is your sting
you shelter me Lord underneath your wings